BIODYNAMICS OF OSTEOPATHY

Phase One

Second Edition

James Jealous D.O.

For more information about Dr. Jealous please visit:
https://BiodynamicsOfOsteopathy.com

BIODYNAMICS OF OSTEOPATHY Phase One

Hardback ISBN: 979-8-2954-6318-1
eBook ISBN: 979-8-2954-6319-8

Editing assistance: Gregory T. Yesensky D.O.

Second Edition 2025

James Jealous D.O. (1943–2021) practiced as an osteopathic physician, teacher and writer for many years. His life's work was to found and develop the specific methodology of Biodynamics of Osteopathy, following the lineage of Dr. A.T. Still and Dr. W.G. Sutherland.

This is one of a series of Biodynamics of Osteopathy books. They grew organically from sets of handouts written by Dr. Jealous and given to students during courses taught by him and his teachers. After many years he collected the handouts together and created individual course manuals, which he added to and rewrote many times. After several more years they evolved further into books.

TABLE OF CONTENTS

OSTEOPATHY IS SERVICE

We use our hands ...

To treat the Whole patient

To listen to the indwelling movements of Life

To treat all levels of illness

To assist in building the patient's functional reserve

To support homeostasis and trophicity by balancing the activity of the autonomic nervous system

To explore "laws not framed by human hands" (Dr. Still and Dr. Sutherland)

To cooperate and communicate with the Laws of Nature (Dr. Wales)

"To find the Health" (Dr. Still)

To get to the treatment plan

To get to the diagnosis

To help establish a point of Rest or Neutral around which the Whole can come to balance

To find Cause

We believe …

We have an innate capacity to heal
The patient functions as a whole
The autonomic nervous system plays a major role in disease and healing
Structure and function are one form of activity
The Divine is indwelling
Life moves beyond death
There is a Constant Movement toward Normal
We are here to Serve Humanity

Normal is …

"A sense of peace and harmony" (Dr. Sutherland)
Ease of motion, without tension
A capacity for Neutral
A sense of Wholeness to Life
The capacity for adaptation, change without compensation.

"Skill is proportionate to one's understanding of normal" (Dr. Still)

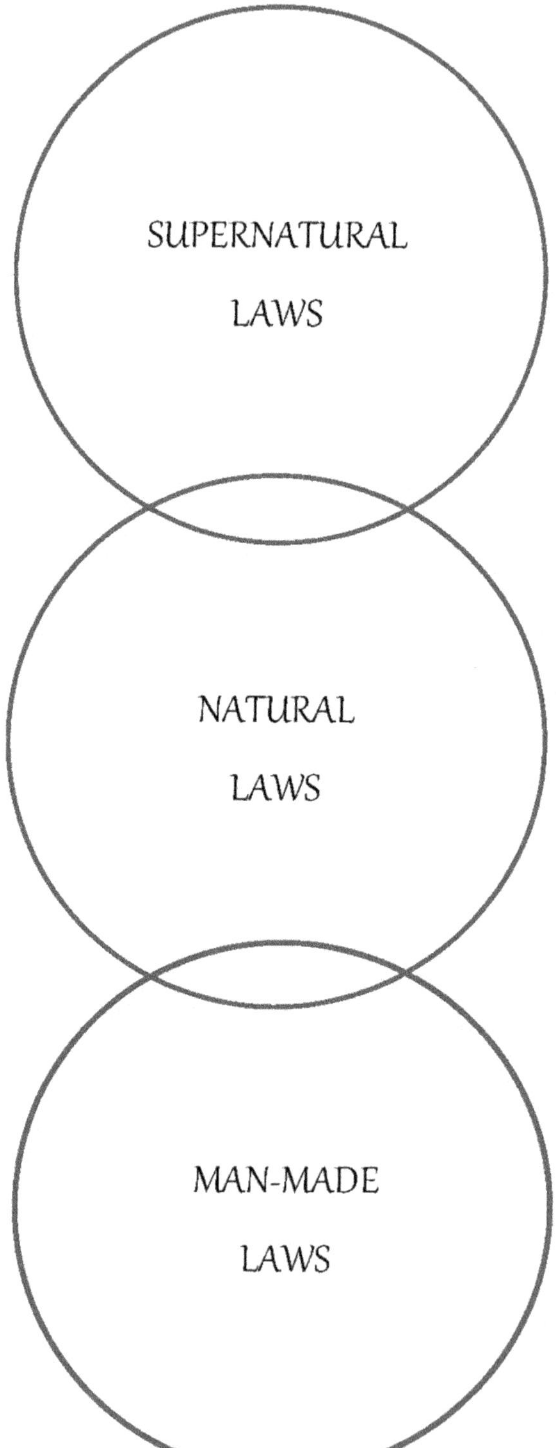
SUPERNATURAL
LAWS
NATURAL
LAWS
MAN-MADE
LAWS

THE THREE CIRCLES

This diagram will help your discernment as you work with the indwelling laws in your patients. The division is based on the teachings of Dr. Still and Dr. Sutherland. The divisions ultimately are not real, as these circles exist as one reality that becomes apparent in later Phases. Understanding what you are feeling helps you cooperate and communicate with the formative and healing forces that are expressed during treatment in the embrace of Primary Respiration. These circles will help you better understand the potency (transmutative power) of what is present and its potential. This information comes into the senses only when they are passive, afferent, and listening, not when a physician's intention is efferent, active, or decisive.

I was trained to communicate and cooperate with natural law as my primary role as an Osteopathic physician. Natural laws are not something most educated persons are aware of instinctually; rather, most tend to "think rationally" about natural laws, which is of no use in an art form such as the general practice of Osteopathy.

We must sense an activity, listen to it, and wait in silence so it can speak to us from its essence. From this communication one begins to partner with the wisdom of the therapeutic forces, which, as we know, are the formative or embryological forces. This communication and cooperation augment the movement of healing.

This profession has a real service to offer in any state of compromised being.

The upper circle is supernatural laws, which are Divine and not influenceable by human will. You will feel unconditional love and many miraculous movements during treatments that arise from this landscape.

The middle circle is natural laws, set in motion by creation and embryonic intelligence. Natural laws can, in general, be manipulated by man, but not to the depth of disrupting the integrated whole. All diseases have, as we know, a natural history, a behavior that in some cases is a predictable pattern ... unless interrupted by supernatural forces that reinstate homeostasis, which is balance in the whole organism.

This happens constantly.

The lower circle is involuting and cannot grow, thus defying natural law.

THE EMERGENCE OF ORIGINALITY

The title of the first manual written for Biodynamics of Osteopathy was "The Emergence of Originality." The title came to me as an image of what a treatment feels like when approached from the laws reflected to us by Primary Respiration.

What emerges in the patient from behind the veil of their illness is a new sense of themselves ... a Wholeness.

Over many years as a primary care physician, I saw remarkable changes in patients as their Original Self (Health) emerged and their sense of well-being flourished. Osteopathic treatment endeavors to bring the patient to the discovery of their own Health. It demands skill, proper thinking, mental discipline, and patience.

As a country doctor in rural Maine, I had the privilege of meeting many self-made individuals who did not "worship" doctors but gave their respect once an individual earned it. Bringing Osteopathy into an environment that had been considered an Allopathic domain for generations was a challenge. But Osteopathy proved itself to both me and the patients. In six months' time, my practice was at capacity, even with five other doctors within twenty-five miles of where I practiced.

Most days began with a twenty-five-mile drive to the hospital to make rounds on inpatients. Hospital care approached by Osteopathy soon turned many nurses into believers as they witnessed the thinking and management of a traditional Osteopath ... from conservative use of medications, to the time spent sitting with patients and families, to the hands-on treatment. People saw a difference when compared to the Allopathic approach practiced by the MDs on the hospital staff.

The Allopathic model and Still's model of healing are very different, and, as one will see if one tries Osteopathy, it will heal many conditions that drugs cannot reach. The difference between Allopathic thinking and Osteopathic thinking is dying in a flurry of status seekers and businessmen who are controlling the practice of medicine for personal gain, leaving the Osteopathic principles out of the educational model in favor of the mass production of physicians, who are losing their creative fire and conscience.

One of the goals of Biodynamics of Osteopathy is to teach Osteopathic thinking in the lineage of Still, Sutherland, and many unheralded DOs who did not compromise the deeply unique and effective methodology of Osteopathy as practiced by primary care physicians.

Be assured that Osteopathy is not a neuromusculoskeletal specialty. It covers much more ground than what is in that specialty. There are many principles that do not begin with the vertebral segments. It is important that one sees what Osteopathy truly is within itself, not as an isolated category.

In Biodynamics we will sense Wholeness as a Reality, hoping it will emerge in ourselves.

The service of Osteopathy creates fertile soil for self-discovery and real education about healing and truth as it applies to the human condition.

The Emergence of Originality is the purpose of life ... to come to a point of balance and peace within oneself. Normal is when "all the fulcrums are synchronized ... and there is peace and harmony" in us (William Garner Sutherland).

From newborns to elders, patients will heal, but ... some do not. In them the capacity for healing and finding themselves "healed" does not depend on curing an illness but rather living in Wholeness ... This truth is not a philosophy but an empirical fact that only someone who practices Osteopathy can witness directly ... human beings are incredible ... your patients will prove this to you ... belief or disbelief is not the issue ... it will be placed before you as an unavoidable fact.

Osteopathy will humble you. You will be awed by truths that will prove to you why Dr. Still became so well known and loved as a physician ... and why this profession was created and why its truths will live on in spite of the modern medical trends toward biochemical medicine, with predetermined formulas leaving the uniqueness of the patient unacknowledged as a central tool in getting well.

Worldwide, there is a tendency to think like MDs, and very few recognize that Thinking Osteopathy is not easy ... "find the Health" ... "treat the whole patient" ... "find Cause," not cause and effect ... "study the laws of nature inside of us" ... listen ... Wait ...

I am not trying to paint a picture of doom, but rather to highlight our heritage and the work that many of us have done and are doing to become more Osteopathic in our hearts ... it is a journey ... Still and his direct students gave us a map ... we should not throw the map away until we have reached our destination.

Osteopathy is a school of medicine. It has a lineage. It is an oral tradition.

We respect all other schools of healing. But we must not become them, or our gift to humanity will perish, as will the passage of the tradition.

Osteopathy is a tree ... there are many branches ... they are all from and part of the Tree ... none are to be pruned away or ignored ... as we grow, the Tree is strengthened by what we give back to the Roots.

Discovering the Original Osteopathy and letting it emerge in your hands and hearts will take great effort—effort not to slip onto the easy road of "cause and effect" mentality ... an effort to free your mind so you can see what is really happening in yourself and the patient ... it will make you work ... and it will prove itself to you, then it will become an inner place of rest forever.

Then it will "speak to you."

You will then feel its voice and its loving hand creating the image you seek ... the Health that Dr. Still saw in the World ... which is Eternal.

BIODYNAMICS: WHAT DOES IT MEAN?

The word "Biodynamic" was chosen for these courses because of parallel discoveries by W. G. Sutherland, D.O., and Erich Blechschmidt, M.D. The word was positioned in medicine by Dr. Blechschmidt. We have extended it to envelop the dynamics of Primary Respiration as expressed by William Sutherland, D.O. The reason for this inclusion into the science of Osteopathy is that Blechschmidt and Sutherland both describe the same principles innate to our creation, growth, and healing. Even though embryology is at the very roots of Osteopathy, no one, to my knowledge, has seen the similarities between the observations of Dr. Blechschmidt and Dr. Sutherland and applied them in practice.

The word "Biodynamic" has a special meaning when seen from the summation of both men's efforts to unveil the movements of life. Both men are recognized as pioneers. Both men, one working with growth and development and the other working with healing through transmutation, described similar processes in the internal activity of protoplasmic fields. When I saw the similarities, I was elated and doubtful, as it seemed almost unimaginable. As I studied further, the parallels were everywhere, unavoidable and precise. The clinical application of these principles in a general practice setting revealed an even greater-than-imagined improvement in clinical outcomes. Today, these principles are widely used in Osteopathic practice worldwide, because they work!

The History

The foundations of Osteopathy are in embryology, which all but a few Osteopaths have forgotten. The embryological segment has become replaced by the vertebral segment. Most Osteopaths are thinking about bony lesions and direct action to relieve "nerve pressure" as the basis of treatment, rather than having a direct awareness of the Indwelling Capacity of Natural Laws to express themselves in a symphony of therapeutic movements.

The role of the autonomic nervous system in disease as a principle based in embryology is being neglected in much of our thinking and educational orientation. The segmentation of the embryo is the foundation of how we should think. Our elders all thought from these principles as they tried to excite or inhibit functions of the autonomics at many levels, including the whole patient's internal milieu.

Osteopathy Is an Applied Art

Will Sutherland was interested in embryology. He encouraged his students to read embryology. He used embryology as the foundation of his work on the extremities in his later years (see "Power Points" in Phase Six). He was grounded in a working knowledge of embryology, as you shall see in this and other commentaries.

My first exposure to embryology was in Kirksville College of Osteopathic Medicine (1965) ... I was spiritually awed by the unfolding process and the mind behind the beauty of growth and development. My anatomy fellowship mentor, Dr. George Snyder, wrote papers on the embryological development of the fascia. We studied embryology and segmentation at Kirksville in order to be more effective at diagnosis and treatment. At the time, Pottinger was the text that we depended on the most, but in recent times, the works of Michael Kuchera, D.O., better serve our purposes in understanding this workable truth.

Later, in 1980, John Harakal, D.O., then the president of the Sutherland Cranial Teaching Foundation (SCTF) in the US, asked me to do a lecture on the development of the central nervous system for the SCTF Basic Course.

As I set forth to review and update my knowledge of the subject, I first went to Dr. Sutherland's writings, reading and rereading "The Tour of the Minnow."

As usual, when one reviews the masters in any tradition, it feels like a "first reading" ... one truly wonders if one ever read it before.

As I read, I ran across the words "lamina terminalis" ... I did not know what it was ... so ... I tried to look it up ... not easily forthcoming. Book after book on anatomy was naked on the topic ... One embryology text showed a picture of the lamina terminalis as the membrane closing the anterior neuropore of the third ventricle during early development. It was obvious that the lamina terminalis was not common knowledge.

How did Sutherland know about this? I do not know, but I suspect he was patient in his observations of involuntary motion ... a task that most DOs would find uninteresting and tedious. He watched without overlaying his ideas on the Mechanism—remember, he was the first to see Primary Respiration in a medical context ... And he had nothing to lead him but his mental freedom.

Sutherland was an Osteopathic thinker and explorer

He discovered what science cannot yet find ... a moving process in the patient that can be appreciated both in diagnosis and treatment, leading his profession into new territory. The motion had a rhythm; he called it Primary Respiration because it was different from thoracic respiration and seemed to be more essential to life. Dr. Sutherland worked and renewed his thinking for nearly sixty years.

Sutherland's conclusion about the sensory experience of Primary Respiration was expressed in a painting created by his wife. It was a house under the sea with all the doors and windows open and the fluid tidal wave passing freely through the house unimpeded. This is a biodynamic picture of an outside extra-genetic force creating and giving life in a precise and perfect manner. It matches the picture one gets from reading Blechschmidt. Blechschmidt had only a microscope to work with; Sutherland had all his senses honed by years of patient Osteopathic observation. The story of how Sutherland progressed in his capacity for observation is important to anyone who wishes to follow his trail and see the things he saw in the internal natural world of his patients. The trail is not well blazed; one must go slow and be exact in understanding the process of divergent observation as opposed to reductionistic mental processes. One important point about Osteopathy and embryology: it is what causes embryology that interests us as much as the patterns of individual parts and their natural history. Why? Because wholeness is one of the first principles. We study the capacity of the Whole and the cause of Wholeness as well as the inverse, the loss of wholeness and the cause of its breakdown.

The First Principle Is Wholeness

Dr. Still was deeply aware on many levels that there is a real wholeness that one can access. This was a reality for him. The tragedy is that many osteopaths think it is philosophy and not fact, therefore never placing it in their sensory experience. The modern osteopathic scholars in America often say that the body is a unit, which paints a lesser picture of a human being by leaving out the patient's soul and spirit. Human beings are embraced in a world that they do not always "sense." As children we do sense this; as adults, ninety-five percent of us are reductionistic and have removed our natural senses from the foreground.

The sensory access to wholeness has been unexplored by our teaching institutions, and yet it is the tool we use all day long in practice. Sutherland and his students were patient observers, who, as Sutherland said, tried to think independently of what they knew. This perceptual stance is one that is fearless, and being so, it finds many moments of awe and beauty. Still had this, my teacher had this ... it is what exposes wholeness and allows the thinking of Osteopathy to be free from its enemy: reductionism and dependence on an Allopathic model in the mind.

This statement is in no way meant to degrade Allopathic medicine but rather to highlight the necessity that justifies our professional uniqueness.

Interestingly, just recently, Dr. Raymond Gasser published a paper on wholeness ... again embryology moved forward, and as it does ... the principles we live by in Osteopathy become better known and appreciated.

At first, I thought the lamina terminalis was just the name of a place, but Sutherland points to it as a place to and from which the central nervous system takes it motion—as a fulcrum. It is a functional pivot and a doorway to the "Sea Around Us."

As I was totally frustrated with the information in "the books" ... I turned to the librarian at the University of New England College of Osteopathic Medicine where I was an off-campus clinical professor of Osteopathic family practice.

After thousands of dollars and months of waiting, thirty or forty articles from all over the world that contained the words "lamina terminalis" arrived in the mail ... most were vague, but one article mentioned that the lamina terminalis was the point where the torus opticus unfolded into a myriad of functions in central nervous system development (see CNS lecture in Phase One). I was aghast.

Sutherland clearly saw the importance of the lamina terminalis as a "fulcrum" for the pattern and power of central nervous system motion, and now we find that his kernel of truth was pregnant. The lamina terminalis was a fulcrum for the growth and development of the central nervous system as well as many other functions (see Phases Three to Six). The story of his clear understanding will come through as we proceed in this commentary.

Will saw the importance of the lamina terminalis, and somehow he knew of its function in the unfolding of life before the science of embryology discovered it.

The first lecture I gave was, for me, exciting news about the wisdom of what Sutherland noticed and how deep this truth was.

Unfortunately, not everyone thought I was brilliant. Some of the board members were certain that I was crazy. There was panic and doubt all directed at me in a flurry of rejection, but ... four physicians stepped into the fire with me and supported what I had found in my reading: Rollin Becker, Robert Fulford, John Harakal, and Jacques Duval ... they literally called off the irritated mass of experts.

I was confused at the frantic response. Some faculty members were so angry at me that they thought I had invented the whole thing ... which of course I had not ... I was following Will's words to the letter.

My interest did not wane. I read and read ... all kinds of strange (to me) articles ... I was seeing, however slowly, the deep connection between the Health as Still taught, Primary Respiration as Sutherland described it in the fluids, and the forces of creation that unfold our inner embryonic world, as Blechschmidt described them.

In another five years I was a real "nut case" ... often dreaming that my embryo was talking to me. I fell in love with the livingness and sweet silence in which all unfolding occurs.

My critics were hard; they clung to the safety of the past and their position as teachers ... At that time I was forty years old. They were thirty years older. Now that I am older, I can understand the critics better ... something Will was confronted with. Most critics are cowards, never directly debating the issues, only commenting in dark corners. The critics have helped me look deeper and harder and have been most helpful in my developing these connections. They have my gratitude for pushing me into clear water.

"A little learning is a dangerous thing; Drink deep, or taste not the Pierian spring" ... This quote is from a poem by Alexander Pope entitled "An Essay on Criticism." It was set in the title page of the first edition of Will's book. The poem is very useful, as it gives insight into the constant rejection Will digested in his easy manner and kindness.

He is a role model one can easily admire for his tolerance and neutrality.

I know I have not said what the use of the term Biodynamic means, but I am getting there ... the story goes on!

As my research into embryology continued, I was directed to Blechschmidt's article in *Symposium on Development of the Basicranium* (National Institutes of Health, 1976) by my childhood neighbor, Frank Willard, Ph.D. All along the way he has been a good critic and generously answered questions as they arose.

I realized I was "out on a limb," alone

I discovered descriptions in embryology that paralleled Sutherland's comments about his observations gleaned from listening to the fluids as they responded to Primary Respiration. These parallels narrowed and met.

There are pictures of the metabolic fields in Blechschmidt's writings; in particular, near the end of the text *Biokinetics and Biodynamics of Human Differentiation* ... These pictures describe forces at work in the metabolic fields ... well ... they are the same as what Sutherland described. The pictures in Magoun's text are exactly the same (pages 100 and 101, third edition of *Osteopathy in the Cranial Field* by Harold Magoun, The Cranial Academy, 1976).

For example, in one of Blechschmidt's figures there are two men inside the fluid field facing each other and pushing toward each other ... in other words, the two men are bringing the metabolic field toward the "center" ... the same as in a CV4 where the forces of the "fluid in the fluid" are brought to a central point creating Neutral ... through which therapeutics become active.

Another picture in Blechschmidt clearly defines a spreading apart of the metabolic field that replicates Sutherland's base spread done with only the gentlest of touch ... this has been called EV4 in the biodynamic model because the Direction of Ease in the fluid field is the opposite of that in a CV4. Other pictures represent what we would call disengagement and opposing physiological activity.

As I saw all this, the light came on ... both of the men, one with a microscope and one with his hands, were watching the same process. It seemed too simple to be true, but there it was. I was a little overwhelmed ... everything stopped ... the partitions came down. The oneness was incomprehensible ... the models of Primary Respiration I had been taught and used for years shattered, and a "breath of something other" entered the shoreline of my little mind.

Intuitively I felt a warmth and admiration for Still and Sutherland ... also, I saw again how long it takes to be aware of nature's laws at work in patients rather than adding laws "framed by human hands." I grew up in that moment ... no more compromise.

Sutherland's perceptual journey was critical for his understanding. He had to change how he worked and how he thought ... the perceptual re-clothing of his awareness was a hard task. He had to rethink his formulations over and over ...

Because of this synthesis, I reread and catalogued all of the perceptual steps I could recognize in the complete text of *Contributions of Thought* by William Garner Sutherland (The Cranial Academy, 1967). The key was the observer changing and being free of bias.

What Is the Word 'Biodynamic' All About ... ?

The premise of indwelling therapeutic forces inside of us came through Still and Sutherland very clearly ... so clearly that many have decided that it is just philosophy.

Sutherland followed Still almost word for word. My whole entry into Osteopathy was because I trusted nature more than politicians or businessmen ... when I read Still, I was sold ... then I applied to Kirksville, announcing to them in my application that I was only applying to one school and, if rejected, I would stay in graduate school until they accepted me ... Recollecting now some fifty years later ... there I was immersed in a sea of truth from many sources ... I was elated ... but there was more.

Sutherland's model of Primary Respiration was "a house under the sea" with all the doors and windows open and the Tide moving through with ease, bringing form, function, and healing.

Blechschmidt's sense of the metabolic fields in embryos was that they were biodynamic; that is, they were an expression of an outside extra-genetic force of creation known only to the embryo ... not scientists, but the embryo ... an ocean that is through us, creating involuntary motions (biokinetics) and self-correcting activities (automatic shifting).

An Ocean ... A House ... Transparency of the Whole to the Creative Forces

As I assimilated these little pieces, years passed, into the early nineties ... but there is more to the question. What is Biodynamics and what is behind the word?

Metabolic fields, whether in embryos or adults, are about the death of the old and the building of the new ...

Metabolic ... catabolic ... anabolic ... in this metabolic fire, what is it that synchronizes the death and growth of form and function? What creates the death and what transmits the boundary of the function that is unfolding?

Metabolism does not happen without a catalyst, and at the most essential level that catalyst is unknown ... Sutherland used an ancient Greek word to describe the metabolic shift ... Transmutation (see Ovid's poem *Metamorphoses*, from the 8th century) ... a complete change ... a change so dramatic that it was akin to a change in species, not genus ... change as a result of transmutation.

Blechschmidt did not have the tools to go as far as Sutherland in this direction

Sutherland's hands became transparent to this Truth. He himself grew into an intimate relationship with the Biodynamic Sea Around Us to the point where he saw through the effects into another fulcrum (cause) ... that could only be called that which lies beyond transmutation ... The Breath of Life ... herein is the power of creation entering the sea, which has the potency to transmute biostasis, the enemy of growth and healing, and reestablish freshness.

These facts may seem poetic, but the facts stand by themselves, unalterable, precise and unerring. A Mystery known only to the innocence that an embryo images to us, but also a concrete fact.

As the Biodynamic model and methodology grew from 1978 to the mid-1990s, many people became interested again in embryology and began to study the unfoldment of life.

I caution the reader to remember that Sutherland went beyond the form into the cause that makes embryology happen ... this is a different study from that of embryological milestones.

Biodynamics is not about forms or formats ... it is about the intimate manifestations of Primary Respiration as a creative and therapeutic force that transmutes the old and carries the image of the new into place. This ability to transmute lies behind all success in treatment, behind all spatial and temporal interfaces that unfold as development and growth occur ... through neutral homeostasis.

The Sea Around Us Is Biodynamic

As yet, embryology has not caught up with Sutherland or Still ...

I do not encourage the study of embryology beyond a point of basic understanding and awe. Rather, study Primary Respiration ... look behind the effects ... what is the cause ... and what are the means of communication with that cause and its intention?

The test of these truths is not in logic but in the clinical advantage they bring to the varieties of suffering a country doctor witnesses ... all patients benefit in many ways from hands that diagnose and treat from these foundations ...

Still called it life, "that slow vivifying force coming forth from God." Sutherland called it Primary Respiration ... It is one.

Biodynamics Means All of This and More ...

Blechschmidt chose the word to make the point that there are extra-genetic forces at work in the creation and the unfolding of embryonic life. Sutherland saw that force at work as transmutation coming from the Sea Around Us ... and ultimately from the Creator. Mix the points of these two men and you will find the word "biodynamic" and its meaning.

There is more than my lifetime can hold, but to those who love Osteopathy, I have written this for you and no one else.

WHAT IS NORMAL RELATIVE TO THE BIODYNAMIC MODEL?

Understanding the development of a function is essential to the answer. Embryology expresses billions of functions; each one emerges from a seed or fulcrum that is present throughout life. To say that "when all the fulcrums are synchronized there will be peace and harmony" is to enter the universal mind that perceives wholeness and not duality. Dr. Sutherland clearly saw the upper circle and this Truth.

Expressions Of Normal Function

1. An ease of motion, tensionless-ness; to feel this in yourself is amazing
2. Natural disengagement, ability to change shape with respirations
3. Synchronization by a Higher Wisdom
4. A relationship with the Whole
5. A capacity to adapt without compensation
6. A capacity to come to rest
7. A capacity to relate to other parts through relationship to the Whole
8. A conscious connection with cause
9. A capacity for distortion and return

Normal is…

"A sense of peace and harmony" (Dr. Sutherland)
An ease of motion, without tension
Being neutral
Wholeness
The capacity for change

"One's skill is proportionate to one's understanding of normal." Why would Dr. Still say this? Normal requires a point of rest. It is through this point of rest, or Neutral, that the organism maintains its integrity as a whole. It is through the point of rest that the indwelling healing forces restore and regenerate function and form. The capability of a function depends upon the function being connected to the perfect blueprint that shapes our embryonic life. This blueprint appears at conception . . . it is called the Embryo, or the Health … the unalterable perfection in each living creation. During the resting phase (neutral), the homeostatic forces (Primary Respiration, thoracic respiration, and the perceptual axis of the immune system) synchronize with the Health to bring the parts into a Single Movement called Wholeness. When this happens, there is a sense of complete transparency to the movement of creation, which is everywhere; this "sense" is called Love. All of these normal activities can be experienced by Osteopaths if they Think Osteopathy. There is a constant movement toward normal; this is called growth. The indwelling magnetic pull toward the Health and Normality is the Health in us moving us toward itself, which is our "higher nature." As Dr. Sutherland said, "This is not an idle dream." As an avid believer in Osteopathy and having seen its benefits in well over 150,000 office visits as a country doctor, I can say that Sutherland's dream was real.

Since 1966 I have traveled this road, and finally I feel ready to participate in Osteopathy as I believe Still envisioned it, to find the Health, the core normality that creates us and heals us, not as a spiritual ideal but as an indwelling capacity to return to the Health.

What is normal? What does that experience feel like? Normal is not an outer appearance or behavior, it is the state of being in the Health through the Tide's healing. Normality is a state that has perceivable tension, an awareness of the flow of love through all of us and knowing that one does not know. It is the sensation of Life in everything ... one becomes like a child. To be an Osteopath has always required courage and commitment, especially today when the Allopathic model is so much a part of one's education.

Biodynamics is designed to cross the bridges and the landscapes that our elders traversed ...

We walk in peace with all Osteopaths, regardless of their bias, and we walk with respect for all healing arts but understand the need to keep Osteopathy as pure as possible. If you work to Think Osteopathy with your heart and hands, it will come true; it will prove the principles to be sound and accurate. Normal is a Wholeness ... this is hidden from the average Osteopath because of the mental orientation to tensions in the lesion during treatment.

Wholeness is a fact, a reality that is easily overlooked. Modern embryologists are just coming to see into this Wholeness as the basis of growth and development. Still spoke about this many years ago (see chapter 1 in Philosophy of Osteopathy, CreateSpace, 2014).

Biodynamics begins with the awareness of this Wholeness. The movement of creation begins as a Wholeness. The embryo unfolds as a single syncytium, as a single drop of protoplasm that becomes diverse. The diversity is growth. It occurs as a singularity expressed from a master blueprint that we call the Health."

We are from one substance, the Breath of Life.

It yields many forms without diminishing itself.

Healing comes from renewal of form from one substance, the Breath of Life.

FORMS

Electromagnetic or Fluid in the Fluid or Potency or Fire

Molecular or Fluid Body or Biochemical

Physical or Mechanical or Tissue

Mind or Supreme Intelligence

Soul

Body

TEACHING BIODYNAMICS OF OSTEOPATHY

The word "Biodynamics" is used in Osteopathy in the same manner as it is expressed in embryology—that is, a force outside the embryo creating the internal events of growth and healing. This almost unbelievable reality is present throughout life and dictates much of the beauty seen during treatments. Drs. Still and Sutherland were deeply affected by this "outside movement" and its internal action observed during the healing process; they called it a supernatural force because of its miraculous clinical results and indifference to human will. This constantly flowing River of Life profoundly affected their perception and skill. They both observed being centered by these forces and were awarded insight as a result of the exchange. This Great River is also called "the Tide" or "the Ocean." They are symbols and, as such, bring us a deeper reality.

You and I will grow deeper into our own true nature if we follow these principles. They are the Osteopathic legacy of this program, which is a direct extension of Dr. Sutherland's private study group (1935–1953). With this understanding of the Primary Respiratory Mechanism, the actual teaching of this work will move in accordance with the flow of the tidal forces mentioned above. As such, we may appear to be disorganized. Our devotion to the biodynamic movements of life has proven to be clinically profound in a general practice setting and just as profound within our own lives.

We are here to serve you and not to clone you into a slave of a belief system. Osteopathy is a journey into the interior of the natural and divine laws that beautifully and silently guide our lives into the stream of our deepest hopes.

The language has been expanding throughout the history of Osteopathy. Definitions fail to penetrate the sensory experience of these phenomena and thus leave one mentally confused. The action that creates the words carries the story of who or what something is. This action becomes clear from "cooperation and communication" with the biodynamic laws of the natural and supernatural worlds, present from the beginning of mankind's search for harmony and Wholeness in his collective life.

Separating your skill from the collective will limit your access to these laws and perhaps frustrate you ... so let's try to follow the moment-to-moment motion of the whole as we find the Breath of Life, the Tide, the River of Life, Primary Respiration, the Mechanism, and other motions that share many different names in our legacy ... the names are symbols; the actual motion, if listened to in the Whole, will reveal its true nature, truth and Joy.

WE USE THE FOLLOWING OSTEOPATHIC GUIDELINES WHEN TEACHING BIODYNAMICS

Find the Health in the participant, not liabilities.

Respect their ability to explore this work without a table-trainer constantly beside them.

Apply principles rather than techniques.

Use questions as a direction for topics.

Allow students to go "with the Tide" during practical sessions, not just the instructions.

FOUNDATIONAL SKILLS FOR OSTEOPATHIC MEDICINE

Wherever or whatever we do as Osteopathic physicians, we carry with us a different foundation than that of other professions. "First, do no harm" is a well-known phrase in medicine and an essential one for living. What does this mean in terms of awareness beyond the words?

When in the presence of a patient, and especially when our hands are engaged in discernment, we should be aware of three basic responsibilities:

First, be aware of the whole patient. This includes body, soul, and spirit. The ease of this comes with maturity as one becomes less involved with the disease itself. This will support healing.

Second, observe the interplay of the autonomic nervous system in the patient with what you are doing, even during history taking. Many people unknowingly have post-traumatic stress and a low threshold in the sympathetic instinctual response. We do not wish to create an imbalance by the use of our attention.

Be invisibly kind.

And lastly, listen to your conscience. One's conscience is not a learned morality or a religious belief, it is an indwelling awareness of a higher wisdom that unites all living things. Osteopathy will put you in touch with your own Health or True Self, which knows the upper and middle circles innately. Do not add pressure to yourself to get results at the expense of the well-being of the patient.

These functions are often lost in modern living and education. You do have an inner balance scale of universal meaning that supersedes man-made laws. This will emerge as you treat the patients and not their diseases ... a virtue indwelling in Life.

PERCEPTUAL STUDIES: DISCERNMENT

The assumption in Osteopathic education that all students perceive in a similar manner is a serious mistake. There are intellectual, intuitive, and instinctual faculties that can dominate one's orientation toward palpation or sensing. There are active hands and passive hands. Neutral hands are usually connected to a deep respect for the Tide, and a dependence on being centered by it usually comes with time if one pursues neutrality. Biomechanics is based on two active hands and a mental schematic overlaid onto the patient. This corrects lesions at the exclusion of the whole patient.

Functional methods are many and diverse; all depend on at least one hand being passive, or listening, not actively palpating. Functional methods look for "ease" in the lesion. The listening hand plays a major role in following and leading the treatment into a "neutral position." This is less efferent than the biomechanical and uses the afferents to pass data from the "listening hand" to the brain, where a moving image is formed. The formed moving image in the mind is very different from the preformed image used in biomechanics that is efferently overlaid on the patient and lacks motion. The end point reaches into the whole directly.

Some students begin with passive, listening hands, and some with active hands; the feedback to the teacher from the two types will be very different on the same patient. This is also true of teachers. To be mentored, one must discern how the teacher is working.

Another category is seen in beginners who are instinctual, usually from aboriginal communities or someone with in-depth training in contemplation (inner stillness). These students are listening, afferently, with all their senses, waiting for Spirit to open them and to bring images into their awareness. Oddly enough, the intellectuals do not see the value of these normal perceptions. Persons with these gifts are often rejected as unstable or subject to "fantasies," when in fact they are inside natural laws. This last group has what may be seen as the "highest level of creative intelligence." They have imagination. Yet many "educated" people narrowly see imagination as a disability … interesting.

Ultimately, if one practices Osteopathy, a variety of perceptual skills converge into fluency. The cause behind the methods comes into the foreground and the divisions are meaningless … but … Which skill do you have naturally? Which needs work? And what is your desired outcome in twenty years? These questions need to be pondered! If you wish, you can try breaking old habits by using some or all of the following practices:

- Learn to "turn the page": Whatever you see, note it in detail, do not reject it, then turn the page, like in a storybook; just turn the page and see what is next, let the story move on, do not hold the images, let them go, and new ones will come in. The key is to see what you see first *in detail*. Don't dive in deep hoping to find treasure; work with a tempo and precision that does not create involuntary changes in the whole.
- Abreaction: This is similar to turning the page, but the intention is more active. See what you see and do not react to it, see it but do not engage with its motion or barrier, stay out of the game, do not let your attention go "there" … A new picture will arise; study it from a distance and do not let the attention get involved. Detach by moving toward the Health away from the temptation to engage the performance (no matter how grand). Pause your mind; empty any sense of a goal. Let images pass by until one centers you and awakens you to its presence.
- Look for something you never saw before: this is very demanding and equally rewarding. Wait until you see something "new."

- Divide your attention between the foreground and the background. Then place 90 percent of your attention on the background.

The squeaky wheel gets no grease; do not let your mind be pulled in by noisy lesions.

MONITORING THE PATIENT DURING TREATMENT

When I treated with Ruby Day, Anne Wales, or Rollin Becker, it was clear that they had a sense of the Whole during the entire treatment. Having the appearance of working locally, their awareness was everywhere as the Whole responded to the Tide.

As we treat, we monitor certain aspects of the patient and begin to see into Wholeness. As we go through the phases, the Whole will become something greater.

First, always divide your attention between the Whole and the part, the Whole receiving the greater part of your attention...85 percent at least.

MONITOR

The local activity

The activity of the Whole

The autonomic nervous system

Your conscience

Always rebalance when finished.

INVOLUNTARY MOTION

The whole functional shape of the organism is breathing with Thoracic Respiration and Primary Respiration. As Osteopaths we can appreciate how the motion of these two breathings, Thoracic and Primary Respiration, comingle and move masses of physiology. This breathing suspends all form and function as it shifts position and physiology to give life in every moment. The fulcrum of origin for respiration shifts constantly as the organism moves, eats, digests, et cetera. Also, this function is then seen as a suspended automatically shifting Wholeness. Sutherland repeatedly describes his observation of this involuntary motion, as many others do. Every time you take a step, read a book, or fall in love, the fulcrums shift and the functional motions shift place.

This picture of normal living movement replaces adynamic gross anatomy as a static picture. This picture is the foundation of Osteopathic medicine and why it is effective in a general practice setting. This event of breathing is a deep physiological principle necessary for health and self-healing processes. The above description is ideal and can be observed in children and really healthy adults, but most often we find these two respirations asynchronous in patients that are coming into our offices daily. So one observes that thoracic and Primary Respiration are separate because they are not in communion with their own health.

Practical

As a practical, observe involuntary motion in the system by listening to and exploring thoracic respiration and Primary Respiration of the clavicle.

Thoracic respiration and the clavicle

Primary respiration and the clavicle

Listening to both at once

REBALANCING IS A VITAL SKILL IN GENERAL PRACTICE

The initial balanced membranous tension (BMT) technique involved direct action, which Sutherland and all his study group abandoned. They were influencing the dura mater to move the bones of the cranium. This then caused reflex nausea and vertigo when the patient sat up. Over the years, principles evolved to prevent and treat these side effects. The method used to influence the bone's repositioning involved using the sac in which the bone was embraced to make the change. The sacs, or layers, of the skull were called meninges. The word "meninges" means membranes and does not refer only to the dura mater but to all the membranes of the cranium. And thus the term "balanced membranous tension" was used to describe the technique.

The key was not to move the bone but its periosteal sac. Take a second and visualize the periosteum and its function of producing bone. The envelope in which the bone rides is its shape-maker. The dura is not periosteum, even though it may appear that way in a dry specimen.

We do not move the dura ... ever ... it is highly populated with nociceptors, and if you have ever seen meningitis, you will remember the severe pain and rigidity that arise from this tissue. So the language itself needs clarification so that the history here can be appreciated and not repeated. Thus BMT is, and is not, a helpful term in a modern setting. The avoidance of using force to make a correction will become simple, easy, and fruitful ... but as Dr. Wales so humbly said, "We cannot give the perfect treatment, so I always check for the need for rebalancing" ... this she did even after seventy years in practice. Her grace as a person was healing.

Post-treatment sympathetic facilitation can occur with anxiety. This almost always follows if one does not listen to the autonomic nervous system while treatment is ongoing.

Again, paying attention to foundational skills as addressed earlier in this manual is vital so as not to stress the physiology. Always check the patient's Wholeness after the treatment. One can accomplish this in many ways.

In each book, we will introduce deeper levels of this awareness.

REBALANCING IN PHASE ONE

Listening to the Whole: does it feel homogenized?

Practical

The Cranial Bowl and the Becker Hold

This practical requires listening with gentle hands.

Rebalancing is only done if the fluid is not working as a single drop.

First, we assess the fluid in the bowl, not the anatomy.

We look for symmetry and fluid motion as a unit.

If asymmetry is present, then we rebalance by going to the central stillness.

Wait.

What happens?

SYNCHRONIZATION BY THE HEALTH

The hallmark of Biodynamics is the intention to be synchronized by the Health. This is an activity that will take you through many landscapes ... it is a journey of a lifetime.

Our first Osteopathic principle is to acknowledge the Health in the patient.

This is a living fact that makes Sutherland's work so beautiful. Our senses will eventually be tuned by the Health, automatically.

When we place our hands on the patient, our first effort must be to synchronize with the Health. We do this easily by becoming aware of the breathing of Primary Respiration. This means that our awareness, consciousness, and perception must be free to do so ... Let your mind settle without controlling it ... then ... sense the breathing and wait. Synchronization, when it is complete, opens the system to a certain kind of stillness that changes your observer and allows observation without disturbing the self-preservational forces of the instinct of the patient.

Anne Wales, a noted and longtime friend of Will Sutherland, stressed this point in her teaching and writing (see page 36, 1953 OCA Journal).

Most people see lesions, the outer layer of what is most superficial in life. Generally, physicians look at patients as diseases, rarely looking for the presence of something that is at the foundation of healing and well-being—the Health. Dr. Still left us with a challenge to find the Health in the patient. We do this in many ways, the first of which is through synchronization with "something healthy" in the patient (i.e., the breathing of Primary Respiration).

As time passes and you relate to the Health in a more direct manner, you will feel the nature of the Health, its essence, and find a shelter. This eternally perfect image of human nature will touch your soul and the lights will come on in your interior world.

A more deeply inherent relationship with the Health is to know it is there whether you can feel it or not. This devotion to truth will open your heart to universal truth and wholeness.

For now, work in a manner that helps your observer be peaceful and patient; allow time for impressions to become evident.

GENERAL SCHEMATIC FOR ANY FUNCTION

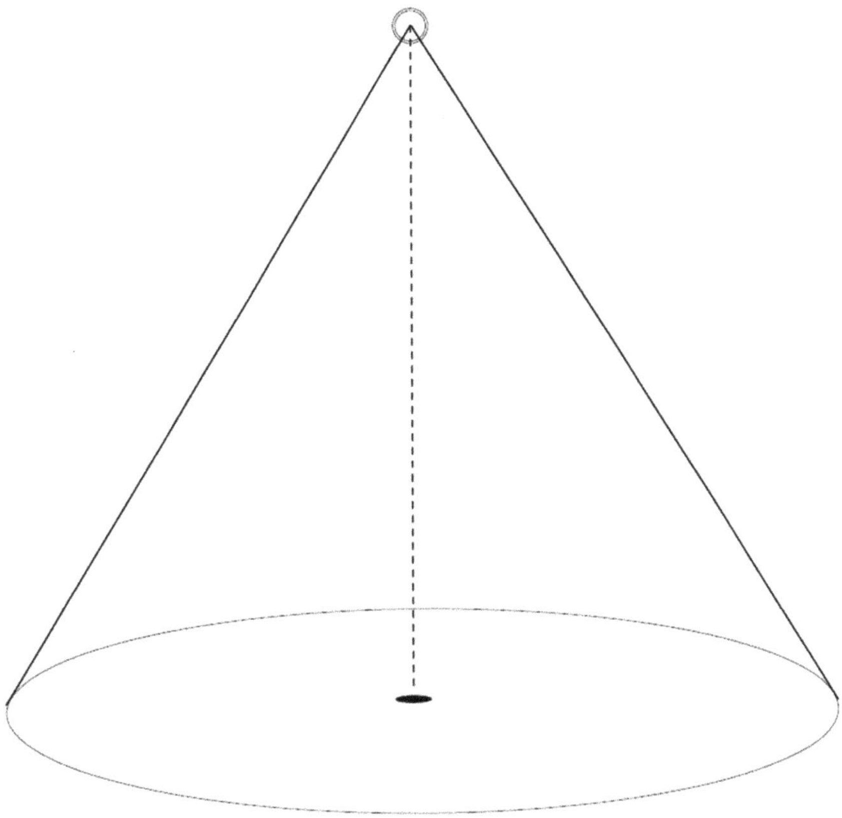

This diagram is about the general principles of embryology and Osteopathy as experienced with "thinking, feeling, seeing, knowing fingers." The instinctual sensory system unadulterated by the rational mind is millions of years old and can perceive motion 1/100 the size of a human hair. We will emphasize instinctual perception during the

Phase courses. Instinctual perception occurs inside an ocean of Silence. Instinct requires silence to perceive subtle movements. In the wilderness, one finds silence as a dominant feature that outweighs sound in its audibility. Inside a patient, we find silence only when homeostasis or balanced fluid interchange is present, or one enters the Health in the perfection of the patient.

The brain trained by man-made laws can only operate in two dimensions, namely afferent/efferent activities that meet synaptic groups formed by education that "react" to impressions with an automatic, noncreative action.

The silence of the instinctual mind is neutral, waiting in a three-dimensional circumference that is miles in diameter. When something moves, there is an imprint that provides images of the origin of the motion, and communication begins. This will become clear as we do the practicals.

The above schematic is what the instincts "see."

The whole image is the function, be it a kidney, liver, or muscle. The shape of the function is what conditions its interior metabolic work. Change the shape and you change the metabolic function.

Shape and function co-emerge at conception from the supernatural world. The idea of a being or function is encapsulated in a seed or primordia, which unfolds over time in growth and development.

The circle at the apex represents the seed or the fulcrum through which motion comes into being and through which the intelligence of the part is intimate with the whole. This is called Primary Respiration. As Primary Respiration breathes, the shape changes; it is a specialized form of inhalation followed by exhalation. This breathing effectuates transmutation, augmentation, and synchronization of the parts with the whole, and an internal change in tone and texture of the metabolic field, called anabolic and catabolic physiology. If perfect, the system reaches homeostasis or balanced rhythmic interchange, where Health is inevitable and a sense of well-being is extraordinary.

The whole functional shape is breathing with Thoracic Respiration as well, so that the two breathings of Thoracic and Primary Respiration comingle, moving all of the physiology. The fulcrum of origin shifts constantly as the organism moves, eats, digests, et cetera. The function is then seen as a suspended automatically shifting wholeness. Sutherland describes all this, as do many others. This picture of normal living movement replaces adynamic gross anatomy as a static picture. Every time you take a step, read a book, or fall in love, the fulcrums shift and the functional motions shift place. This picture is the foundation of Osteopathic medicine and why it is effective in a general practice setting. Turn your head to the left and every cell in your body moves.

DIAGRAM OF A FUNCTIONAL FIELD WITH EASE OF MOTION

Neutral State is Ease of Motion

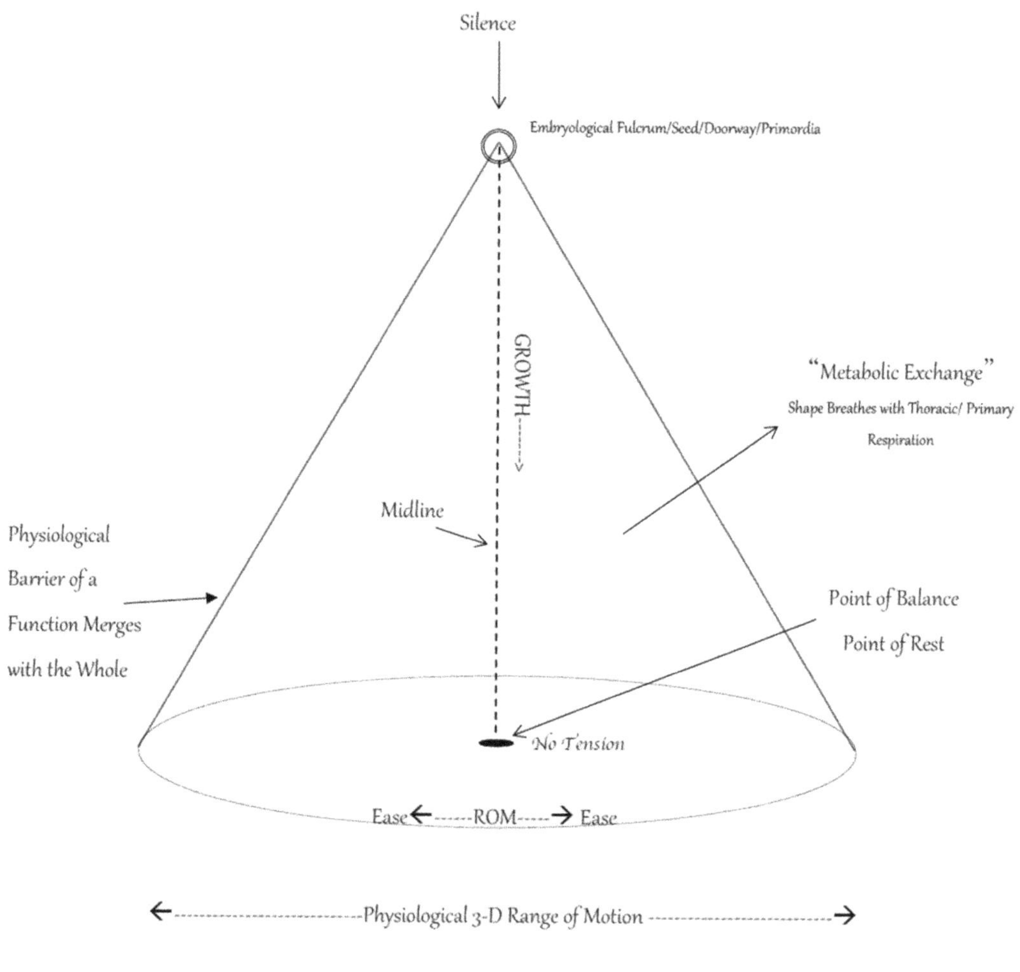

THE OSTEOPATHIC LESION

Herein lies a great mystery of indwelling strength.

Imagine an Intelligence that is in everything, that protects the Whole by moving stress into a form that isolates it and then beginning to transmute it back into its original state. Such is healing ... the science of healing. Imagine further, if you will, a bag of living fluid shaped like the person and containing all forms of energy known and unknown. It is embraced by the soul and transparent to the Beauty of Eternity. This very special person spans a world from embryos to angels. If all I say seems a bit much, well, it is truth incarnate, not philosophy. If you study science, you will come here, but better yet, treat thousands as a primary care Osteopath and see for yourself that this description is not overstated.

When stress exceeds the functional reserve of the patient, the stress imprints the living elastic fluid with a geometric shape ... the shape of a lesion field. This shape is in the Fluid Body but out of proportion with the whole, so it moves differently with thoracic respiration, with formative forces, and with the motion of the body in time. These lesions lack proper flow in many channels. The resultant chemistry is hypoxic, static, and acidotic ... this can make the fluid feel like tissue and tissue feel hardened. The formative forces reunite to "correct the lesion" but only if there is the reserve to energize the process, and if the lesion field can lose some rigidity and become neutral.

The Osteopath assists this process.

There are many approaches. We will discuss them, because over the years I have noticed that practitioners have inherited techniques from their teachers. For example, the variety of BMTs reflects no absolute motif. This of course means that one must be creative within the model they are given. There should never be a debate over who is right, because everyone must work with their own temperament, and modifications often bring out the best in oneself.

We will now look at some schematics that are designed to make you see Osteopathy as a unique science that engages the Health in the lesion field. This reality is rare in any human effort, that is, to see Health as omnipresent and relate to it. An Osteopathic lesion is not between bones. It is an area of disfunction containing all physiological compartments. It is not an orthopedic event. It is not a dislocation. It is not subluxation. These are common misnomers and need to be recognized in any discretionary diagnosis. Somatic dysfunction is a play on words that fails to be scientifically accurate in clinical practice and removes one's observer from details. So ... before we risk a definition, let's look at the lesion as it has lived down through the ages.

Normal is an expression of a higher Mind. Embryology recognizes this Mystery. Every function, be it tissue, chemical, or electronic, emerges as a syncytium form ... a seed or primordium. In literally a flash, the perfect matrix is imprinted and the whole future laid out in its pattern of development. This takes no time at all. The function has a shape usually containing tissue, physiology, and electromagnetic features. The shape of the function *is* the function ... change the shape, change the function. Knowing shapes is called functional anatomy. Shapes are constantly breathing ... they are alive and as such must be renewed on a regular basis.

The shape, as I said, is key to its success as a part of the syncytium. Let's begin with the physiological shape and its emergence in the Embryo, realizing that genetics can alter the shape only so much. A nose will be a nose, a kidney a kidney, even if altered within certain parameters. The limits of this discussion will end here. The treatment of genetic deformities is another topic.

Diagram of Lesion Field

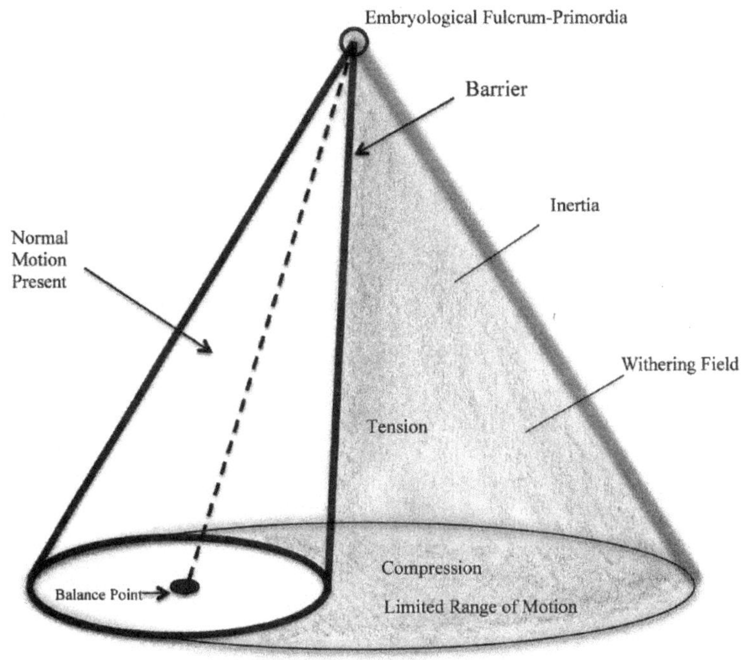

Inhalation Phase of Primary Respiration

Internal Disengagement
Synchronization
Augmentation
Transmutation
Transparency

THE LESION FIELD SCHEMATIC

It is said that an osteopathic lesion is a form of restricted motion within the normal range of motion of a function. The personal relationship to a lesion varies from Osteopath to Osteopath.

A lesion is named for its retained motion, not its inertia. This is commonly misunderstood. The dysfunction is named by its health; this is very Osteopathic. One should ask why seeing a lesion as a healthy expression is useful Osteopathic thinking.

If we compare the normal schematic with the lesion field drawing, we can see normal motion on the left-hand side of the lesion field. The motion of the normal in the diagram is quite large compared with the retained motion in the lesion field. Notice that the whole process of lesioning is inside the range of motion of normal and does not break the barrier ... if it did, you would have an orthopedic event: subluxation, dislocation, compound fracture, et cetera.

Try to settle into the reality of an osteopathic lesion being an intelligent function with retained healthy motion.

If we look at the right-hand side of the lesion field, we see inertia, compression, loss of motion, restriction, asymmetry... most Osteopaths relate to this side of the lesion and attempt to overcome the restrictions.

In functional technique, we begin with the motion in the lesion field that is found through motion testing and go in the Direction of Ease.

The motion present in the lesion field is retained from the normal functional motion present before lesioning. This motion is the name of the lesion used in communication with others ... So a "sphenoid high right" lesion means that this movement is the Direction of Ease exposed during motion testing. This is a profound truth: healing is not a war between normal and abnormal but a continuum of normal until the lesion is transmuted by the healing forces … which are the Health and the parenting forces of the normal function.

In the Biodynamic Method we do not motion test. Rather, we listen to the inhalation and exhalation of Primary Respiration in the Whole and then divide our attention to include the lesion field and observe what kind of motion is expressed during the inhalation phase. Then we synchronize with that motion. A treatment process begins that takes us to neutral in the local lesion field, where we wait for a continuing therapeutic process guided by the Tide that will extend the Neutral into the whole patient.

APPLICATION OF THE BIODYNAMIC METHOD

Practical

Check the whole patient, the autonomic nervous system, and your ease of mind.

Define the boundaries of the lesion field by listening afferently.

Divide your attention and notice the breathing of Primary Respiration.

Observe the shape of the motion present in the lesion field during inhalation.

Synchronize with the motion present ... this is automatic.

Now begins a therapeutic process.

When a lesion forms, it is not randomly produced, even though it may appear "accidental." Actually, a lesion is organized by the Health. The Health works within the physiologic range of motion to make definite, distinct disproportion possible. Lesions obey natural laws, and as such follow lines of "natural" deformity up to the point of resolution or destruction.

The lesion catches the Whole person in the web of its form. So when a lesion patterns, one lesions as a unit of function and not segmentally. The lesion is only in the Whole. This concept must be grasped in order to appreciate the forces of Health.

THE PATIENT'S NEUTRAL

The word "neutral" began to be used by Sutherland as a metaphor relating to a standard-shift automobile. Today, few people understand the value of the term in clinical observation. The history of the word goes back to Fryette's description of the laws of mechanics where neutral was a normal state of readiness for engagement by voluntary or involuntary forces in movement. Neutral sounds like a flaccid state but is anything but. It is a state of readiness that waits to perform when influenced by a direction from outside itself. Think about this natural state spiritually ... one waits in silence for the initiation of action from a higher mind. It is not a place of laxity but one of readiness, joy, and expectation. Neutral is *not engaged but ready to be engaged* by natural forces. You may find synonyms for Neutral that are meaningful, but today let's see if we can recognize this state in a patient.

Neutral will occur in the whole patient. There will be a sense of a single tone or texture that lingers throughout. To reach this state the patient needs time, while your listening hands appreciate the presence of the Health or a pervasive Stillness. The patient will slowly and then more rapidly approach Neutral while you give your attention to the indwelling Health. Feeling the Health is not your task but rather acknowledging its presence (seen or unseen). Waiting is a skill that takes no effort, because the landscape where you wait is refreshing.

Some patients cannot get to neutral, and so we help them ...
this is a Phase Two topic.

THE PATIENT'S NEUTRAL (CONTINUED)

Neutral is a state of Neutrality. It is very alive and Dynamic. The knowledge of this must come from experiencing this state in yourself and in patients. It has a history in our profession that goes back to Still, who did not use the word, but once you are familiar with the nature of Neutrality and Neutral you will "see" it in Still's words.

I first became aware of this teaching in the Functional Methods teaching in Kirksville in 1967. Later I read more in Bill Johnston's text. Additionally, there was an article from the New England Functional Study Group around 1953 by Dr. Bowles entitled "The Dynamic Neutral." Karen Gajda, D.O., found references by Dr. Fryette as early as 1916. Dr. Sutherland was well aware of this state, which he sometimes called Neutral and sometimes Idling. If you have studied the CV4 in Sutherland's writing, you may have realized that he employed the CV4 to allow Neutral to manifest in the whole patient. This Wholeness is the First Principle of Osteopathy and is the doorway to Primary Respiration, in an extremely healing process.

The Neutral state in the whole patient is the landscape through which the Tide can work using its Supreme Wisdom to guide healing in the same manner in which it creates and unfolds us as embryos.

What does neutral feel like? To the patient it feels serenely empty and restful. A productive Neutral will shift the consciousness as well as the physiology ... BUT ... not if the patient's observer is watching the treatment. I say this because in Phase One many D.O.s want to track what is happening to them as they are treated on the tables. This ultimately is a good thing gone bad.

Neutral feels homogenized.

When milk is homogenized, it becomes one substance, not layered.

In a Neutral state, the patient has no gross anatomy. They feel like a "single drop." Their whole being is like a gel. The gel-like state is not water, it is protoplasm. The gel can become more rarefied, and if it does it becomes more transparent to the Movement of Life as Still described it and as Sutherland witnessed.

Once this state is entered, it can last several minutes ... the clinician waits for it to express its steadiness and quiet. It is different from a Stillpoint. This level of discernment will come as you do more treatments.

The important task for us now is to learn to wait and let the neutral ripen. When the neutral is complete, there will be a new rate that is slower than the pre-neutral rate. We will work with this in every Phase, so do not rush to understand it.

All of these activities are part of the indwelling therapeutic forces that hallmark Osteopathy as a unique and great profession. When we profess to acknowledge and communicate with these laws of healing ... we mean it not as an ideology ... it is a living truth that will really heal and reorganize the whole patient.

We will study how to wait peacefully as we watch the Tide move the patient toward neutrality, after we simply synchronize with the Health.

Neutrality is a state of active receptivity to the healing potency of Primary Respiration. It is a peaceful wholeness expressed by the physiology when all the parts come to a relative or absolute state of rest and return to a relationship with the Health that created the wholeness.

It is a place with specific characteristics that the skilled Osteopath can interpret in a general practice setting.

THE PATIENT'S NEUTRAL

Practical

This practical is about Synchronization, Waiting, Observing your Mental Habits and the "work" done by the patient as they "move" into Neutral.

Sit at the feet ... Synchronize with something beautiful ... Listen to the inhalation and exhalation of Primary Respiration ... Wait ... Observe the patient's movement toward Neutral; do not help. Observe any tendency you have to interact with things that happen. There are pauses ... Stillpoints ... and finally, a Neutral.

Neutral is a state of wholeness, fluid homogenization and breathing at a steady rate ...

THE ALCHEMICAL NEUTRAL

I. A Point of Balance

Healing requires a new pattern to transpose the pattern of disease. Osteopathy in the cranial field acknowledges the potency of the Breath of Life as a dynamic resource in transmuting patterns of dysfunction. In order to follow the intention of this Breath of Life as it prioritizes and interfaces within the patient, one must be able to recognize the point at which the whole individual is receptive. This is a sensory impression of a point of balance, a state of receptivity in the patient. We call it the patient's neutral.

II. Neutral

The point at which a direct response to the Tidal forces is possible; a point of balance in the reciprocal tensions of the whole that is free to shift with Primary Respiration.

III. The Patient's Neutral

A point of balance unique to the moment and the individual through which the Tidal forces can act to regenerate function. This point of balance is collective, a function of the Whole, an integrated tone of body, soul, and spirit. Through this "neutral," the priority and intention of the Breath of Life is able to permeate and "work" with as little unresolved tension (in the patient) as possible. Infrequently, due to disassociation of the soul-body-spirit unity, the entire treatment may be the reinstitution of a Neutral. The Neutral tone can be sensed as a homogeneity of all forces, as a single texture that emerges throughout the

Whole patient. At this point, the patient is most responsive to the Breath of Life.

IV. The Alchemical Nature of the Neutral

The point of balance described above has a sense of density and being. This collective texture may vary from lead to liquid to light and also from visit to visit. It is always the point where the individual is free to respond and be shifted by the Tidal forces. It is a point of receptivity and nurturing and may be consciously appreciated by the patient. Here, at the tone, transformation is possible. The variations of resonance are infinite, so we never "automatically" know this point. The density of the neutral does not condition healing. It is the point of maximum receptivity. Remember, the Breath of Life does not proportion its wealth, but through this fulcral point delivers 100 percent of life to each person. The tones are different but not in the scale of recognition. The tone is set by the proportions of the body-soul-spirit mixed into a single reciprocal tension, the tone for that moment. The reciprocal tensions meet in a collective harmonic, a chord of notes that merges into one single tone.

V. The Value of Knowing the "Note" of the Alchemical Neutral

The tone is used as a reference point for understanding the intention of the Tide, which is very clear when this unified state of balance is evident.

The tone is also used to determine the amount of force or "tone" used by the clinician when a technique is applied. For example, the application of CV4 is much easier and the end point realized earlier if the neutral tone is applied to the system; that is, we match any force upon the system to the "note."

Respect for the patient's neutral will deepen our awareness of the remarkably precise and wise integration of life that is created by laws "not framed by human hands" (W. G. Sutherland). Here we see the deep organized relationship that each person has with the Great Hands of Life and how each of us has a special and willful consciousness of the genuine, essential Whole and the "note" of resonance. Our hands, guided by the Neutral of our patients, will allow us to visit this enlightening relationship between each unique individual in a moment of creation. It is for healing that the Neutral is there, so that the Breath of Life can "move us" as a unit, not as a mechanical device. You see, our ideas die in the face of this reality. Our idea of who the patient is and what they need dies in the Unexpected Precision at the interface of life and evolution.

Another value of patiently appreciating the neutral zone is markedly fewer treatment reactions. This is a result of remaining harmonically in touch with the innate tone of the patient. End points are clearer. Overtreatment is avoided because the Neutral and the Breath of Life are respected. One will easily appreciate this benefit after several applications of this principle. The primary tone and site of treatment cannot be established through information from lesions. We tend to idealize the treatment process and treat using the most potent form of application we are familiar with (i.e., potency, fluid, et cetera). One will see that the idealization of potency and depth are ideas we superimposed on the patient's system.

The neutral will define all of the elements in the equation that summates the Whole and integrates it perfectly with the Tide's intention.

Please, remember not to mistake fluid drive for the Tide itself; this can lead to confusion!

During the therapeutic process, one keeps the "Neutral tone" in mind and stays on that note in all relationships to the forces present or introduced. The Breath of Life relates to the whole person through this "tone" or alchemical neutral, a point where one can shift in response to the Will of Life.

VI. The Recognition of the Neutral

The prerequisite to recognizing the patient's Neutral is to not react to any motion or fluid activity until the Neutral emerges. One remains Still and Observant and Waits, knowing that all activity will come to a pause, the neutral tone will be evident, and then a rate of approximately 2½ cycles per minute will emerge. The neutral emerges as a homogenized state where fluid, potency, and tissue are not discernible as separate densities; only the unit of the whole at its point of balance for this moment is evident. It is a point where disengagement and healing occur in direct response to the Tide. Understanding the Tidal intention at this point requires perceptual skill that is covered in a different discussion; however, this information can readily be applied to any Osteopathic treatment.

VII. Exceptions

The neutral state will emerge in 90 percent of patients. However, if the neutral does not appear after long observation and normalization of sympathetic/parasympathetic balance, then one must consider disassociation within the Soul-Body-Spirit relationship. This usually results from injuries involving loss of consciousness or psychological terror. In these cases, a gentle, soft, patient EV4 on the fluid to open the longitudinal fluctuation and reestablish midline response to the fluid can begin the healing process, which in these cases is to reestablish the cohesive function of the Neutral. The Whole has been disturbed at a very deep level and needs to rebuild its unity and perceptual integrity.

VIII. The Physician's Neutral

Finding one's own state of neutral requires deep appreciation and respect for one's own suffering, acceptance of the unresolved, and a surrender to the Love of the Breath of Life. Patience in a quiet, natural setting will potentiate this discovery. My own practice is to take time each day, at a specific time, and wait for my neutral to appear. Sometimes another pair of hands appears.

IX. The Stillpoint

At the stillpoint, the patient will consciously perceive the moving Stillness only if the neutral has been realized.

DYNAMIC NEUTRAL , A BRIDGE

As one of the original founders of the New England Academy of Applied Osteopathy, Charles H. Bowles D.O. served as its education director from 1952 to 1956. This is a quote from a short article written by him to explain a phase of development for Harold Hoover D.O. Dr. Bowles wrote it especially for the Academy of Applied Osteopathy 1969 Yearbook, and dedicated it to H. V. Hoover, D.O.

> Harold Valentine Hoover (1940s) used to talk very much about "dynamic neutral."
> ... a manipulative positioning that was guided by dynamic neural clues at the palpating fingertips could establish a normal self-maintaining state of dynamic neutral. In other words, here was a new non-traumatic and accurately controlled way of relieving the structural stress and strain of the "osteopathic lesion." Dynamic neutral is a state in which tissues find themselves when the motion of the structure they serve is free, unrestricted, and within the range of normal physiological limits. The term dynamic means that the structure is moving, is in a condition of living dynamics, the term neutral means that the action and reaction of the serving tissues stay in normal, or neutral, limits during that motion. ...
> ... the restricted motion found between two mal-aligned skeletal units need not lie wholly in a locked or semi locked articulation. There are neural mechanisms at work in the positions of a skeletal unit within the overall motion pattern of its neighbors ...

INTRAOSSEOUS MOTION

This beautiful movement occurs as an expression of transmutation.

This discovery by Dr. Sutherland changed his whole view of the cranial work. His understanding of the Breathing of the Cranium shifted from a rigid model onto a landscape of "Every Drop knows the Tide." Every drop of life in every cell is breathing, and he felt it. This syncytium was moving as a single cell. He had crossed the perceptual barrier between the middle and upper circles. Wholeness was real. Bones are metabolically dynamic. They are breathing and changing shape. They have intraosseous motion. The periosteum extrudes the shape and produces the cells. The formative embryological forces carried by Primary Respiration tempo the rate of growth and development as well as renewal and/or healing. Repair and remolding are carried on by the Fluid Body but only if neutral or a tension-free status is inherently reached by the lesion field. All this is what Osteopathy brings to the world, the engagement of indwelling therapeutic forces by listening with a silent mind. The beauty you will see in the clinic will forever expand into a greater skill. The clinical results will follow in a wake of unexpected Mystery. The technique is simple, the discipline stable. During inhalation and exhalation of Primary Respiration the bones transmute, change shape as well as density.

Imagine you took a milk bottle from the refrigerator, sat down with it at a table, and had both hands around it, just waiting while you awoke to the task ... in this pause the bottle became very warm and started contracting and expanding ... instead of mental shock, you actually felt joy, until your intellect kicked in and told you you were crazy. It was just your imagination. This is how your discovery will go forward ... with moments of childlike innocence. This makes our profession a natural science as Still described it. Truth needs to find us because we are broken in our perception. Sutherland and many others have led us here to the beautiful and refreshing landscape.

The sutures were a topic of great inquiry. The first theory that lasted a long time (and may still be around) was that the dura mater moved the cranial base into flexion/extension with no shape change in the bones and that the base moved the remaining cranial bones, including the sacrum, through a core dural attachment. The sutures were interdigitating gears that transferred motion from one area to another. This model became cloudy when one realized that the sutures had no gears in children and that the individual bones, as well as all tissue, have individual motion as an intimate response to the Tide in a three-dimensional shape shift.

Eventually, the model shifted to a more complete picture as the fluid and the fluid in the fluid were described in detail. This material will enter our hands every day many times. Your witness will bring you images in even more precise tones and textures. For now, do not believe what you read; just listen during the practicals to what you feel. Sharing that as a group will create a very large picture of motion. This is how we grow, from listening with our hands and not looking to the "book" as the last word. Properly skilled Osteopaths do not need to argue about what is true ... it is really necessary to leave what we know today as "once upon a time" and begin again with a fresh mind. Having an image that men have constructed, in the face of the supernatural, needs built-in room for human contradictions. Only know what you now see as what serves the patient ... why? Because the Tide creates the image in a manner that allows you to participate in a world that eclipses your awareness to serve the whole. The creative forces are intimate in every moment of the patient's life from conception and create a specific healing process ...

sounds good, why are we all not well? ... It requires neutral in the whole in order to materialize ... so we try to help.

Practical

Sutures Open ... Bones Breathe

These are handholds that I find useful ... eventually the Tide will mold your hands.

The Original Vault Hold

The Becker Hold

The mm Mercury in the Fluid Body

The Whole Cranium

Three Individual Bones

First Third / Second Third / Last Third

Rebalance by Listening to the Whole (nonspecific)

THE DYNAMICS OF GROWTH AND ADULT INVOLUNTARY MOTIONS

"I have been mistaken and tried to do the wrong thing. I have found it was not in harmony with Nature's ways. Last week and all my life, I gave noxious poisonous drugs to get an effect, when the force borne in us, if unobstructed in blood streams and nerve courses within the body, would have done what was needed, just as it did to bring the infant to full grown maturity."

A. T. Still, D.O.

Dr. Still notices a deeply important truth: that the forces of growth and development are still present in the adult as healing forces. This is the premise of the Biodynamic Method that arose through a study of embryology and Sutherland's Fluid Body dynamics in 1982. Modern science has verified these realities in its awakening to processes like neuroplasticity. As early as 1998, it was stated in the *Journal of Cognitive Neuroscience* that embryological forces are present in the adult brain as healing forces.

As a result of thousands of hours of observation, we have been able to appreciate these facts in our patients and engage these forces in treatment. Ultimately, Osteopathy is about listening to involuntary motion(s) in the patient and arriving at treatment through an understanding of the nature of indwelling therapeutic forces, without adding force or intentions of our own.

We will begin with balanced membranous tension and work toward deeper realities. BUT ... our understanding of anatomy is going to pass into a new light.

THE BIODYNAMIC AND BIOMECHANICAL PRINCIPLES: A COMPARISON

1. The biomechanical method, or direct action, reflects Sutherland's earlier ideas and principles. The biodynamic ideas and principles reflect Sutherland's later guidance by the Breath of Life.
2. The biomechanical model recognized five phenomena. The biodynamic model stresses one phenomenon with a plurality of effects, none of which are part of the five phenomena as expressed in Magoun or the early Sutherland writings.
3. The theoretical axes of motion for the bones is a central theme in the biomechanical model. The biodynamic model stresses a four-dimensional motion in "every drop" of our being.
4. The Mechanism as a word is loosely applied to the effects in the biomechanical model, whereas for traditional Osteopathy, the word Mechanism was equated with a supernatural order originating from the Breath of Life. Biodynamics has continued this orientation.
5. In the biomechanical method, the "innate forces" are not specifically defined; it is general or philosophical language. In the biodynamic model, every effort is made to communicate and specifically define the innate forces by direct sensory awareness of their natures.
6. The biomechanical model teaches the cranial rhythmic impulse as the primary expression of Primary Respiration. The biodynamic model sees rates as effects and the Breath of Life as the primary expression.
7. The only rate identified in the biomechanical model is 8–14 cycles

per minute. In biodynamics, the base rate in busy adults is 2–3 cycles per minute, and no rate in healthy children.

8. Disengagement is applied by the operator in the biomechanical model. In the biodynamic model, disengagement occurs with the potency of the Tide, not a force coming from the operator's hands.
9. Biomechanics sees perception as automatic, based on palpation, whereas the biodynamic model experiences perception as an active, passive, and then neutral process, eventually guided by the "Deity that centers us."
10. The biomechanical model teaches that lesions are between bones, whereas the biodynamic model sees lesions as a wholeness.
11. Biomechanics does not, as biodynamics does, recognize a biologically active midline.
12. In biodynamics, the personal skill of the student is used as a starting point for teaching, whereas in the biomechanical model the practical sessions are not individualized but constructed around specific outcomes that must be pursued.
13. In the biomechanical model, individual bony position is the key indicator for normal. In the biodynamic model, the indicator for normal is the degree of neutral in the whole.
14. In the biomechanical model, the connective tissue is the means of addressing the relationship of parts, whereas in biodynamics the continuity of relationship is in the relationship of the parts to the Whole, the Whole being a Neutral substance.
15. In biomechanics, the focus is on finding lesions and reducing them; in biodynamics, the goal is created by the Tide and its intention. The operator discovers new diagnostics.
16. The idea of neutral is not in the biomechanical model.
17. In biodynamics, no motion testing is done as it is in biomechanics.
18. "Osseous motion is in the whole bone, inside and out." This biodynamic principle is not pursued in biomechanics.

19. In biomechanics, exaggeration of a lesion means going directly into the direction of the barrier. In biodynamics, exaggeration follows the Direction of Ease, as described by Sutherland.
20. In biomechanics, lesions of the face and vault are approached through the base. Biodynamics follows the automatic shifting of the therapeutic forces within the bone.
21. In biomechanics, it is possible to have a lesion with no motion … not so in biodynamics.
22. Biodynamics stresses thinking beyond the known, to Think Osteopathy. Biomechanics is a rationalization process where the theory dictates one's rationale.
23. Biomechanics stresses the dural sickles as prime movers of the cranial base. Biodynamics does not. The motion is an effect of the Whole under the transmutative forces of the Potency of the Tide (Breath of Life).
24. Biomechanics states that there are three sickles. Biodynamics sees the dura as a sac with fourteen duplications that are of concern to the discerning Osteopath.
25. The biomechanical model has not changed since 1943. The biodynamic model is growing … this is the nature of man's relationship with nature.
26. Biodynamics watches the Tide direct itself, whereas biomechanics teaches directing the Tide.
27. Love is a real expression of life. Divine love has an essential role in the process of biodynamic practice. Biomechanics does not mention love.
28. In the biomechanical model, children's symptoms are related to bony entrapments occurring via specific cranial nerves … biodynamics views the symptoms as a lesion in the metabolic forces of the Fluid Body as a whole.

THE STEPPING STONES

Phase One in Biodynamics of Osteopathy is a stepping stone across a river into the landscape of Primary Respiration.

It is important not to isolate these new principles from the stepping stones that brought you to this particular place in your professional life ... there are more stepping stones ahead, all leading to the integration of your hands and thinking into communication with the Indwelling Laws of Healing as recognized by Dr. Still in the foundation of a new profession.

The actual act of becoming an Osteopath takes time because one's mind is not aligned with the perceptual task required. We have ideas like "treat the whole patient." Well, anyone can like the idea and believe in it, but the reality escapes the senses unless they are trained ... in other words, you must experience the "wholeness of the patient" much beyond any idea you may fortunately possess. The skill of seeing into a truth directly is one of Still's recurrent reminders to his listeners.

Dr. Sutherland's perceptual odyssey is revealing ... he was trained by Still and his writings reflect sixty years of continuous perceptual change. I have cataloged his transitions in "The Sutherland Perceptual Odyssey."

Sutherland worked hard, tested Nature; she spoke back, and he listened and changed his thinking and principles of treatment ... he created the stepping stones for us to follow ... Imagine discovering a whole new therapeutic power called Primary Respiration. I cannot impress on you, no matter how much I try, what this task must have required of his body, soul, and spirit.

The profession never openly supported him, but many general practitioners did. Taking his work home and applying it, they began to reach cures otherwise impossible. Most of his students are gone, but while they lived, they created a legacy by mentoring interested Osteopaths. You may choose to follow that legacy or not, but here you will meet much of it, and it is what we adhere to.

As we make our crossing, I will do my best to relate stories of these women and men who framed the education that is now here with us. Osteopathy is an Art. Out of the Art comes the Science. The science comes from repeated observation of nature's therapeutics and laws.

OSTEOPATHY IS AN ORAL TRADITION

Tradition in craftsmanship is a hands-on learning process. It requires an apprenticeship. Apprenticeship is not in the classroom. It is in the craftsman's place of work. The student must want to spend time learning the principles of the art; then, in time, they begin to learn the craft in their own shop, returning to the teacher when they need more input … This is often a lifetime relationship.

Dr. Sutherland had apprentices from 1935 until his death. For over twenty years he groomed and studied with more than fifty practitioners.

Mentoring is vital to the continuity of Osteopathy.

THE PRINCIPLES OF MIND, MATTER, AND MOTION

1. The body is a living composite of bioelectric, biomolecular, and biomechanical principles all interchangeable and mutually transmutational. In a normal state they are inseparable, as they are a living substance.
2. Involuntary motion occurs everywhere in the whole.
3. Involuntary motions are automatically shifting around suspended fulcrums that are points of power, organization, and reciprocal balance for the part as an expression of the whole.
4. The pattern of motion is established within the fulcrums by biodynamic generative forces. This force is called by us the Breath of Life, and it designs and moves all forms of life at the most fundamental level.
5. All motion is spatially oriented to a midline.
6. The spatial dynamics of life are eternal for the given form.
7. Location and motion are changed by stress.
8. Normal is not positional. It is functional.
9. Motion cannot be destroyed, only condensed.
10. Asynchronous motion precedes disease.
11. To reestablish motion, one must find motion that is already in balance with the Breath of Life.
12. All motions, fulcrums, and spatial dynamics should, under ideal circumstances, be synchronized and reciprocally balanced in their tensions.
13. Lesions are universal within the individual, not local, isolated events.
14. Protoplasm has an internal rate of 100-second cycles, as demonstrated

under the microscope. The motion moves in one direction for 50 seconds, then reverses. This is the base rate for the natural world when scrutinized. Rollin Becker observed this in patients and pointed us toward this realization, which was appreciated at a later time, around 1988.

15. $E = MC^2$.

WHAT IS YOUR RELATIONSHIP WITH THE LESION?

If you are conditioned by modern Osteopathic education, you may have an allopathic view of an Osteopathic lesion and not really know it.

A lesion is not an enemy to be conquered by forceful means. The lesion itself is an intelligent living process, not a disorganized tissue field separate from the whole.

We believe that anatomy exists in the manner we read about in books or see on a cadaver; this adynamic view of structure is archaic and false. A living person does not have anatomy as a separate tissue complex.

What was Dr. Still's view of anatomy? ... We often hear about structural, anatomical lesions, but not in the manner in which Still and his subsequent students sensed living tissue. All of his students thought osteopathy would point us toward a more scientific and complete awareness of what is under our hands.

PHILOSOPHY OF OSTEOPATHY

Recommended reading: *Philosophy of Osteopathy* by Andrew Taylor Still, especially pages 16 to 19. Here is a brief quote, where Dr. Still emphasizes the importance of anatomy:

> You want some standard author on descriptive anatomy in which you learn the form and places of all bones, the place and uses of the ligaments, the muscles, and all that belong to the soft parts. ... all parts through which blood and other fluids are conducted. ... another room or branch of anatomy called physiology, ... how the blood and other fluids of life are produced, and the channels through which this fluid is conducted to the heart and lungs for purity and other qualifying processes, previous to entering the heart for general circulation to nourish and sustain the whole human body. I want to impress upon you that this is as much a part of anatomy as a wing is a part of a chicken. ... in the room of histology you are still studying anatomy and ... to the room of elementary chemistry ... the laws of association of substances that you can better understand what has been told you in the physiology room, which is only a branch of anatomy ... to the room of the clinics, ... with both the normal and abnormal human body, which is only a continuation of the study of anatomy.

THE SUTHERLAND PERCEPTUAL ODYSSEY

During the span of an incredible lifetime, William Sutherland devoted his energies to the activities of Primary Respiration. His model began with a dynamo in the central nervous system creating motion that moved the dura mater, which then mechanically fluctuated the cerebrospinal fluid and moved the cranial base bones at the basisphenoid-basiocciput articulation. From this primary motion at the base, involuntary motion was transferred by "gearing mechanisms" to the face and the vault. And by dura mater in the spinal cord, called the "core-link," the motion was transferred to the sacrum.

Sutherland changed his model to that of the whole system being moved by the Breath of Life ... this change from Mechanics to Transmutation as the abiding principle took from 1898 to 1948. For fifty years he labored to communicate and cooperate with the indwelling laws of Health, as had his teacher, Dr. Still. As Sutherland labored, he became a student of the Breath of Life and gave up the popular Newtonian mindset of his day. His final years found him "not knowing" how the Will of Primary Respiration worked; he said to Anne Wales in 1954, when asked what moves the fluids, "I do not know," a statement of humility from a master Osteopath, who became a light for all those who followed his explorations ... may he rest eternally in peace.

Recommended reading: *Contributions of Thought* by Dr. Sutherland. We can track his perceptual shifts.

The Chronology of His Progress

Birth: 1873. In 1898, he was twenty-five years old and a student at Kirksville with Dr. Still. One day, while looking at a mounted disarticulated skull, he noticed that the squamous temporal-parietal bone articulation looked like the gills of a fish; if you noticed this you would agree. Will had the thought that "the skull could be breathing," that the sutures could be for a breathing mechanism. Later, I learned that the skull he observed was mounted underwater; this raises some questions as to what Dr. Still was up to!

1939, age fifty-six. He introduces the cranial concept and states that the cranial bones can lesion and that they could be reduced (repositioned). Techniques were very forceful, sometimes using bands around the head. Having studied balanced ligamentous tension with Dr. Still, he was looking for the agency that could move the bones. He conceived the idea that the dura mater was a ligament that could move the cranial bones. Lesions were seen as "exaggerations" of normal positions. He pulled on the dura mater as a lever system that he used to correct bony lesions. The model was conceptual, a line of thinking used by Still to correct vertebral lesions but without force. The articulation between basisphenoid and basiocciput was seen as a vertebral articulation because it is a synchondrosis. There is cartilage between the bones, somewhat like a disc, only with no nucleus. He did not listen to tissue forces as a guide to his activity ... he noted the "malposition and used force to restore the position to normal." This was to change a lot as he began to listen to the Mechanism.

1936, sixty-three years old ... now thirty-eight years into his exploration. He begins teaching a small group (five of my mentors were in this group). He observes intraosseous motion; he sees "the ethmoid breathing." He describes central nervous system motion as coiling and uncoiling. The bones are still moved by the dura. The reciprocal tension membrane is conceptualized. The vault and the face are described as secondary motions. The temporal is described as rotating but also undulating. The core-link between occiput and sacrum is introduced as the cause of involuntary sacral motion. Forceful technique continues. The RTM is seen as causing fluid fluctuation. Standing postural techniques are introduced. There is no mention of potency, fluid drive, or indirect action as yet.

1942, sixty-nine years old ... forty-one years of observation. He mentions "Fluid Lesions." He notices that if the fluid locks up, then the bones lock up. He is still using force (bands) to resist fluid fluctuations to get Idling. No rates are mentioned in all these years. Undulation is mentioned again. He speaks of the Spark of Life as the animating force of Primary Respiration. He begins to use patient cooperation and breath augmentation during treatment.

1943, seventy years old ... forty-two years of research. He mentions the Breath of Life for the first time, as the Supreme Force that creates the Spark that results in Primary Respiration and its effects. He begins to observe activities without using force, listening.

1944, seventy-one years old ... forty-three years of research. RTM language begins to form. The Bird is described. Motion of the ventricles is explored. Neutral begins to enter as his technique becomes indirect.

1948, seventy-five years old ... major changes. CV4 is approached without bandages, and he applies much less force. Idling and Neutral are mentioned. Potency is isolated as a specific sensation. Transmutation is appreciated. Diagnosis and treatment occur by the Tide. Softness, gentleness, stops motion testing. He directs the potency through the fluids. He understands the Intelligence of Primary Respiration as Divine and sees the Breath of Life release a lesion. He states, "This is not an idle dream." Reverence becomes part of the treatment. Stillpoints begin to be mentioned. He feels the Tide in a dying patient. "Get as far away from your physical touch as possible." He discovers that what happened in 1898 was a Divine Inspiration.

1950, seventy-seven years old ... forty-nine years of observation of natural laws. One one-thousandth of an inch is vital. He describes ignition, power, and flight of the Bird around the third ventricle and the thalamus as a center of power.

1951, seventy-eight years old ... fifty years. Liquid light is described. The space in between forms gains his attention (see Schooley in the 1953 *OCA Journal*). He feels the Breath of Life passing through the fluid. Pauses become important, vital to successful treatment. "Every drop knows the Tide." He sees the fluid as a battery fluid. He struggles with students wanting to do mechanics. The power of the Tide is infinite.

1954, Will passes at eighty-one years of age. He devoted his life to what he did not know, may God bless him even more.

AXIOMS

*Interosseous motion is not mechanical (i.e., non-axial), but a multidimensional motion.

*Osseous motion is a direct response to the Tide and its influence on every drop and every cell.

*The motion of the Reciprocal Tension Membrane limits motion into a physiological range that fulfills the tissue needs.

*The bones translate along the lines of shape created by the Tide ... the Whole is breathing in the Breath of Life and is shaped by its intention.

*Bones transmute and change density during Primary Respiration. There are no biomechanics creating motion. For example, the occipital bone breathes most dramatically on its transverse axis across the lateral angles, not on its midline base.

*Intraosseous motion is the precursor to successful interosseous motion.

*Protoplasm is like a pool from which all functions emerge, including the Soul.

*Bones form inside membrane, membrane being protoplasm. All these compartments are at different levels of cellular density.

*Sensing intraosseous motion is more revealing if one's hands are positioned relative to the forces of the Tide rather than any lesion or distortion.

*Cranial motion is not a sequential event; all motion occurs simultaneously as a response to Primary Respiration.

*During transmutation, heat is produced and can be observed to crescendo from the initiation to the end of the inhalation phase of Primary Respiration.

*Paradoxical motion is common, which means that the shape change is exhalation during the inhalation phase of Primary Respiration.

* Midline contains many locations or positions; the position will determine the shape and function of the metabolism. If we change the position of something, then we change its structure and its function. A human being that can function in whatever place they find themselves is considered mentally stable. Mental health is the ability to change position without compensation.

*Remolding of a bone is accomplished by listening to the Tide and not by directing one's own forces at the distortion.

*The sinuses and venous blood are moved by the motions generated by the Tide, not by mechanical levers in the osseous system.

*The design of the embryo is eternal.

*During the inhalation and exhalation of Primary Respiration, the fulcrum shifts its position.

THE PHYSIOLOGY OF A LESION, TISSUE FORCES

The word "lesion" probably makes you think of a diseased state, and possibly you have been trained to feel a lesion as a form of somatic dysfunction that has as its characteristics asymmetry, restrictions, and abnormal tones and textures. Perhaps you may even feel a lesion as inertia or a compression.

The word lesion comes from the Latin "to injure" ... an injured area, be it somatic or biochemical ...When we think about lesions in the above manner, they have no relationship to the Health ...

But

An Osteopathic Lesion is different ... an Osteopathic Lesion is a form of motion, not inertia ... an Osteopathic Lesion is named by its motion ... how strange to call a disease by its healthy aspect! This hallmarks the functional aspect of the "lesion field." This is one thing that makes Osteopathy so different from the allopathic model ...

As you mature, this uniqueness will be central to your relationship with your patients and yourself.

The injured part is seen through its Health.

The lesion is a form of restricted motion, but that motion is normal within itself, i.e., healthy.

Motion is the central feature of the lesion, and that motion is the lesion's doorway to interfacing with therapeutic agencies indwelling in each of us. The fact that we can help heal ourselves because of this motion is not underscored enough in our thinking.

The lesion is named by its Health and can be healed by the Indwelling Therapeutic Forces.

No other profession that I am aware of sees into this truth ... what kind of thinking uncovered something so meaningful?

Let's see what Sutherland reports from his teacher, Dr. Still ...

"In technic we endeavor to follow Dr. Still's methods. That is getting to the point of release (neutral) with no jerking, then allowing the natural agencies to return the bones to the normal relations and position."

"What are the natural agencies? The ligaments, not the muscles, are the natural agencies for this purpose of correcting the relationships and positions at joints."

"Dr. Still's application of the technic is the gentle exaggeration of the lesion that allows the natural agencies to draw the bones into place."

"Dr. Still has taken my hand in his and allowed me to feel the lesion as it was being exaggerated and then as the natural agencies pulled the bones back into place."

"There is a reason for applying that technic in the cranial mechanism."

"The difference between spinal technic and cranial technic is the difference between an automobile mechanic and a watchmaker."

"We do not force anything into place in the reduction of a lesion."

"We have something more potent than our own force working always in the patient toward the direction of normal."

W. G. Sutherland, *Contributions of Thought*, commentary 1944, Des Moines, Iowa

Again, in the book *A Manual of Cranial Technique* (The Cranial Academy, 1995) prepared by Rebecca and Howard Lippincott and approved by W. G. Sutherland, we find more information about the use of "exaggeration" of the lesion (page 1):

Question: When do we use direct action and when do we exaggerate the lesion?

Answer (by WGS): "Direct Action is contraindicated whenever it is possible to exaggerate the lesion (its motion)."

Exaggeration technic sounds, at first hearing, like a technic that increases the tension, that moves into the barrier, into the inertia—but it is exactly the opposite! Our difficulty with the words is from our thinking allopathically (against the lesion).

A lesion is a form of motion, and when the permitted motion is exaggerated then there comes a release (Neutral), then the Indwelling Therapeutic Forces make a correction …

The indwelling capacity to heal is foundational to Osteopathic thinking … Sutherland and the Lippincotts followed a particular thread of activity that was direct from Still … There were many others that followed this line … but not all … some used direct force on the cranium and did not heed Sutherland's warnings (see remaining text in *A Manual of Cranial Technique*) … more later.

The whole of both commentaries above assumes that your education has prepared you to interface with these words and understand them … this is rare today.

A lesion is a "field of activity" … A lesion field has a variety of attributes … a withering field, asymmetry, restriction, barrier, tension and tone changes, textural changes; it covers an area not just between bones but crossing anatomical planes of function. It has somatic, neural, and visceral influences and compensatory activities from minor to major … Among all this is a healthy motion … it may not be the first thing you notice, but if you motion test the segments you will find motion that has an easy direction … In an endeavor to follow Dr. Still, we exaggerate the "ease" in the lesion field … this is called indirect technic because we do not directly take the lesion back to normal but follow the motion that releases the lesion field; it reaches a place of declining tension until it is at Rest ... i.e., Neutral ... then the real treatment is performed by the Indwelling Therapeutic Forces (ligaments, fluid, and potency) ... The agency that comes to meet the point of rest accomplished by the Direction of Ease depends on the type of neutral established by the Osteopath ... tissue neutral, fluid neutral, neutral segmental, neutral regional, neutral systemic, or Neutral in the Whole, which is the place where Biodynamics begins and interfaces with the agency of Primary Respiration.

The more you work from this perspective, the more you will see into Sutherland's writings ... (not so with Magoun, who liked direct action and re-edited the first edition of Osteopathy in the Cranial Field after Sutherland passed).

I recommend the following texts:
Philosophy of Osteopathy, A. T. Still (chapter 1)
Contributions of Thought, William Sutherland
Teachings in the Science of Osteopathy, William Sutherland
The First Edition of Osteopathy in the Cranial Field, Harold Magoun, approved by William Sutherland
A Manual of Cranial Technique, Howard and Rebecca Lippincott, approved by William Sutherland

LESIONS ARE ORGANIZED BY THE HEALTH.

Let's continue, just a little, to reinforce the mental attitude that is core to Osteopathic thinking.

"Your skill is proportionate to your understanding of normal." (A. T. Still). Still does not say your understanding of disease.

Understanding normal patterns means understanding the pattern of a function when it is at rest. For example, a muscle at rest feels like a bag of fluid ... because, at rest, it is a "bag of fluid" ... this sensation of rest and ease is a determinant for your end point, not the posture of the bony relationships ... thus, Still says that anatomy is not just gross biomechanical activity but rather is gross anatomy, histology, physiology, chemistry, and the flow of vital functions ... he also relates normal to Wholeness (see chapter 1, Philosophy of Osteopathy).

The place of normal is a place of Rest (Neutral, Idling); at the place of rest the waste products are recycled, the chemistry altered, the autonomic nervous system retuned, trophicity restored, the psyche disarmed, the spinal cord defacilitated, and the immune system is able to make clear decisions (loss of synaptic noise).

This point of Rest is not "seen" when force is applied to the lesion.

I am not saying that high velocity, low amplitude (HVLA) is a force-oriented technic, because many practitioners understand that the rest point in the joint needs to be met before any correction is made ... but many do not.

When we understand the importance of normal and its meaning, then the movement of any given treatment will be toward a greater understanding of normal, because we have developed a "sense" of normal ... this separates the skilled from the less skilled clinicians ... but it also is information that Allopaths completely overlook in their treatment attitudes ... we are a unique profession.

Lesions, then, are distortions of normal patterns of function. Something forces the function beyond its normal capacity, in either increased or decreased tone (range of motion) ... This is true in diabetes and in somatic dysfunction ... If the physiological limits are exceeded, the blood sugar rises or the tissue tension rises—all the same process.

If the harming influence is too extreme, the system may break or die ... and artificial means of support may be needed ... insulin or orthopedic appliance ... this is Osteopathy.

We create a healing environment by creating a place of rest, neutrality ... a place within the center of the range of motion ... the balance point ... In diabetes we lower the blood sugar with understanding, diet, exercise, and treatment that brings rest to the Whole. In somatic dysfunctions we do the same.

Skill involves thinking and feeling and knowing during the treatment process ... not the blind use of force.

Lesions are created by forces that repattern normal function. The forces that generate the lesion "drive it" in a certain direction.

When we find the Direction of Ease in the lesion, it is often in the direction of the insult.

The Direction of Ease is, oddly enough, not toward normal positioning until after the Neutral is established by "exaggeration" of the lesion.

Fluid Body lesions often will go in a similar direction, then after Neutral the corrective forces (Thoracic or Primary Respiration) take it toward normal via transmutation ... tissue then follows the fluid, over a number of days as it reestablishes its natural range of activity.

RECOMMENDED READING

W. G. Sutherland, *Contributions of Thought*, The Cranial Academy, 1967.

W. G. Sutherland, *Teachings in the Science of Osteopathy*, Rudra Press, 1990.

H. Magoun, *Osteopathy in the Cranial Field, First Edition*, The Cranial Academy, 1997.

E. Blechschmidt, *The Beginnings of Human Life*, Springer, 1977.

E. Blechschmidt and R. Gasser, *Biokinetics and Biodynamics of Human Differentiation*, North Atlantic Books, 2012.

E. Blechschmidt, *The Ontogenetic Basis of Human Anatomy*, North Atlantic Books, 2004.

R. DeHaan and U. Heinrich, *Organogenesis*, Holt, Rinehart and Winston, 1965.

J. Opitz, "The Developmental Field Concept in Clinical Genetics," *The Journal of Pediatrics* 101, no. 5 (Nov. 1982): 805-809.

A. Pischinger, *The Extracellular Matrix and Ground Regulation*, North Atlantic Books, 2007.

Seifriz, W., *Protoplasm of a Slime Mold* (Search on YouTube), *Protoplasm*, and *A Symposium on the Structure of Protoplasm*

REBALANCING

Rebalancing is a tool that everyone should understand and be able to use.

Rebalancing is a principle that was taught by Dr. Sutherland, Dr. Becker, Dr. Day, and Dr. Wales. Drs. Day and Wales taught it to me, and I have used rebalancing in a variety of forms since 1976.

During my training at Kirksville, we were all admonished to be able to manage the side effects of any therapy we employed. We spent as much time exploring how and why side effects occur as we did understanding the nature of the treatment employed. The outcome of this balanced study was a greater understanding of the laws of nature and how clinicians or remedies, creating side effects, can insult these laws and hurt the patient.

Biodynamics stresses this principle! It has been rejected by many Osteopathic educators at the ultimate expense of the patient. I believe it should be taught in all schools and courses.

A greater understanding of normal physiological mechanisms will come from observing a system when it is thrown out of balance by a treatment and by restoring balance using the principles we will teach.

Rebalancing Will Be Addressed in All the Phases.

Rebalancing is precise and requires that one does not become anxious about the untoward symptoms that the patient is expressing. Be calm and quietly apply the corrective measure, then wait and see if the system can self-correct once given the opportunity to rebalance; most times Wholeness will be reestablished. Be calm ... this mental state is necessary for you to have a precise sensory awareness.

Dr. Wales and Dr. Sutherland began rebalancing patients because their patients would get some or all of the symptoms listed below from a cranial treatment:

Nausea, vomiting, vertigo, disequilibrium, pain, sympathetic discharge, fainting (catatonia), emotional fragility, symptom aggravation.

Sutherland recognized that direct action was not the best method of treatment... he clearly changed the amount of force used during treatment until he was just an observer.

THE PREVENTION OF SIDE EFFECTS

Prevention of side effects occurs from the moment the patient enters the treatment room and there is a level of peacefulness (an atmosphere) and tranquility in the air.

During Treatment One Should Monitor the Following Activities:

The whole patient ... a sense of wholeness does not include the part, even though one may be working on a local problem. The quality of Wholeness should increase during history, examination, and treatment. If it diminishes, this is a red flag that something has insulted the patient's overall health. This is vital to the functional reserve in the patient. A sense of wholeness does not include structure.

The tension in Zone A ... the overall somatic tension should be declining as the treatment proceeds.

The autonomic nervous system ... facilitation in the autonomics should be steadily declining as the treatment proceeds. There are local, or segmental, facilitations and central facilitations. One should know if the changes occurring are local or systemic, i.e., segmental or brainstem. Any increase in facilitation should be addressed immediately by rebalancing.

Zone B ... should reveal a steady transmutation toward Neutral.

Your Conscience ... follow your indwelling sense of participation. Your conscience will alert you if you exceed your individual gifts. Do not do something because someone has given you a technique. A technique is a dangerous tool if one is interested in the Wholeness of the patient. We follow the principles of treatment and monitor the feedback as described above.

Today we will teach rebalancing from a historical lineage, but I believe rebalancing through the Fluid Body will be the most useful in preparation for Phase Two.

Rebalancing neuromuscular activity at the craniovertebral junction

There is a ring of muscles that circles the craniovertebral junction. This ring of muscles is part of the oculo-vestibular-cephalic mechanism. The ring functions as one muscle when adapting to postural or autonomic stress. Ruby Day told me that they address this during rebalancing because the conscious and vegetative functions of the CNS meet here—the point being that the brain and spinal cord have different interfaces with life and can desynchronize. Please review all of the intrinsic muscles of the craniovertebral junction at your convenience.

REBALANCING: CRANIOVERTEBRAL RING

Rebalancing is an act of humility. When Dr. Wales was 105 years old, she was still rebalancing every patient.

What does that mean?

It means that after the treatment, you can listen to the patient with your hands, and you see if the whole patient is relatively homogenized… so that you are not feeling a lesion. Rebalancing means that at the end of the treatment, the patient should be neutral.

They started giving these cranial treatments, and they got into the fluids and the tissues and they overtreated. It is very easy to overtreat. Patients can get off the table with dizziness, palpitations, autonomic storms, et cetera.

So a lot of people were saying that if you didn't get side effects, you weren't giving a treatment. But Dr. Sutherland didn't feel that way, and all of my teachers did rebalancing.

I think that Dr. Becker was doing rebalancing all the time when he was treating. He was always watching from this really quiet place. And if the patient started to experience any kind of disharmonic movement in their system, he would have to balance his relationship with the Mechanism. So ultimately, the rebalancing will be done as you treat, and in a lot of people rebalancing is the first treatment that we give them. They come in, they are kind of nervous, all stirred up, so we do rebalancing … they feel good … they might get into a total neutral.

So at the end of your treatments, you feel the patient. There shouldn't be anything happening. The whole patient should be moving like a single drop of water. They should be resting; they should be calm.

Sometimes at the end of the treatment, there is a little vibration. As Dr. Wales would tell us, "We leave our footprints in there without knowing it."

All rebalancing, for now, has to do with the craniovertebral junction.

What Is the Craniovertebral Junction?

–It is suboccipital, and there are muscles there.

–Structures in the area include the foramen magnum, condyles of the occiput, and atlas (Dr. Wales would say they looked like bedroom slippers).

–It's where the base of the brain meets the spinal cord; why rebalance here?

This is the junction between the vegetative and cognitive functions in the patient, between the brain and the spinal cord.

You find disruptions between the brain and the spinal cord in whiplashes and brain injuries that go undiagnosed all the time. One of the things we want to be thinking about is to really refine the diagnostics of closed head injury and whiplash. And really get a feel for these muscles.

What Are the Muscles?

Draw a circle ... that is one muscle. All of these muscles at the craniovertebral junction function like one muscle.

Why would we have one muscle? They don't function independently of each other ... they function as a unit.

So see if you can move rectus lateralis, spinous process, atlas, jugular process, occiput. See if you can move that muscle without moving any other muscle in your body. So if you try to side bend right and you move your lateral rectus, what happens if you go too far? Your quadratus lumborum starts to move. Why, if you side bend your atlas, would your quadratus start to move? And who is telling your quadratus lumborum?

When people have whiplashes or strokes, this whole system gets knocked out.

So we have one muscle here; it looks like a circle. Where is the center point? It's in the center; where is that? It doesn't have an anatomical location. It's a function.

When we rebalance it, we are going to feel this circle of muscles as a single muscle, and we are going to find its balance point, and then we are going to wait. You tell me what happens.

We have the anterior rectus muscle. There are two of them, one on the right side and one on the left side. When you whiplash, unless it is perfectly symmetrical, one of them is going to get injured, and the other one is not going to be injured so much. So I ask the patient to close their eyes and look at the ceiling, look straight ahead, and then look down. When you look down, you are going to feel your anterior rectus as your head goes into a very slight flexion. That is what you are going to check for in your patients when you check this ring of muscles to see if it's injured. Because if you miss that, a lot of patients will have residual disequilibrium. Not vertigo, not dizziness—disequilibrium. So they will start to move, and the ring of muscles is not functioning as a unit.

So one muscle goes faster than another, and they start to recruit differently. Often people have vertigo from a whiplash, and it starts to go away, but they are left with this residual disequilibrium.

If I asked you to close your eyes and look down to the floor and to your right side, that would start your lateral rectus. And I would have the patient doing this.

If you ask the patient on the table to close their eyes and look down while you go to the anterior rectus, and you feel this movement to the right, that means they are strong on the right and weak on the left. They have an injury of the anterior rectus that is still there.

The muscle can be normal after an injury, say six months later, but it is desynchronized, even after it heals. So if your diagnosis is correct, then one treatment—rebalancing with the muscles—and the next day their disequilibrium will be gone if the diagnosis is correct.

The muscles recover quickly because they have healed up. But the sensory motor cortex is not synchronized.

They are still recruiting, even though the muscle is fine.

The Muscles in This Area: anterior rectus, rectus lateralis, rectus posterior major, rectus posterior minor, obliques

The oblique muscles function like rotators. So what happens when you try to turn your head? Turn your head slightly; what is the next muscle to move in your whole body? In other words, how is your brain set up? You start to rotate your eyes to the right and the next movement is that your knees are going to start to rotate.

You'll feel the condyles of the femur rotating on the tibial plateaus.

When you evaluate these muscles, have the patient make these really fine movements with their eyes. If they move their eyes to the left and nothing happens, that means that the whole rotator system on the left is delayed. So it is out of sync and you have disequilibrium, but they don't have vertigo.

To evaluate, position the patient without a pillow and with their head neutral, and have them close their eyes. Look down, look up, look right, look left. Don't go too fast. See if they start to recruit or if the muscle actually works by itself.

Then, if you want to rebalance them, you've got to be at the craniovertebral junction. So your finger pad is on the occiput and the nail is on the atlas, and the midline of your finger is on the space in between. We are efferent, listen ... space in between ... at the seam. Once I arrive at my destination and I become efferent, then I can start listening.

What Am I Listening To?

I am listening to this circle, to all these muscles as if they were one. And I am going to the Stillness at the center.

Where do you think these muscles begin embryologically?

Growth and development occur from that center point as a point of orientation. This center point is not in an anatomical or neurological location. But it is the center point for the oculo-vestibular-cephalic reflex and the recovery of function of this one circular muscle. Like a joystick, it can rotate.

You can do the evaluation first. Locate the seam between the atlas and the occiput. Anyone with experience is going to come and put their hands on the patient's feet and they are going to move the AO joint from the feet so that they can tell if they are in the right space. If I put too much force in the feet, you'll feel me move your fulcrum into the head. If I don't put enough pressure, you're going to feel the fulcrum at C2 or C3. But if I put just enough pressure so that I get right into that ring, I land right in that fulcrum and I sit. You're going to feel an increase in your perceptual awareness of the Whole movement of the circle.

So the most important thing is to get ourselves in the right spot. This is called rebalancing. This is the first kind of rebalancing that Dr. Wales tried.

She actually used the back part of her fingernail to move the atlas and the pad of the finger to move the occiput, and she would disengage the craniovertebral junction and let it come to a balance point. We've modified it a little bit, as people misinterpreted it as direct action, which it didn't feel like when she did it.

THE CIRCLE OF THE CRANIOVERTEBRAL JUNCTION

Study the intrinsic muscles of the cranial base: rectus capitis anterior and posterior (major and minor) and oblique, lateral rectus, intertransversarii, longus colli, longus capitis. Sense these as a single muscle with a ring shape.

Find the Direction of Ease in millimeters of motion without recruiting any other muscles such as the splenius capitis, et al.

Move in the Direction of Ease until the sensation of balance in the ring muscle matches the air in the room.

Wait ... until thoracic respiration moves into the ring space that is balanced ... and begins to move the tissue. A series of deepening balance points will precede the final point of ease before there is involuntary motion.

Watch for the following:

–the autonomics should be finding a point of de-facilitation.

–the Whole Patient should be improving ... becoming more neutral.

–your conscience should be agreeing with your actions.

The Long Axis Disengagement of the Cranial Base

Dr. Sutherland demonstrated this approach to his private study group. The idea behind it is, again, a de-facilitation of the brainstem/brain interface. The principle is long axis disengagement done softly with no sense of barrier ... one waits ... the longitudinal fluctuation rises up from the pelvis into the cranium ... the stress declines. This was used even in severe cases where vomiting was occurring ... it was successful. As the study group realized that direct action was not the proper approach, they became more oriented to ease and fluid. Ruby said that Will taught this around 1940 to her group, who became his teaching assistants.

Rebalancing Through the Fluid Body from the Cranium

This is an approach that has been developed along with the Biodynamic principles. It uses the Becker hold. I will describe this in detail during the practical.

We will hold the cranial bowl as if it was a bowl of water. One then waits and listens with the hands. Is the water in and through the bowl still, calm, and balanced, or is there turbulence? If so, then how much? Can you determine Cause ... Once it is established that rebalancing is indicated, then one proceeds to listen with the hands to the stillness related to the fluid, rather than observing the motion(s).

Without augmenting any phenomena, by waiting with the stillness, the waters calm down, become still ... and then begin to breathe rhythmically, expressing a response to the inhalation and exhalation of Primary Respiration.

This return of normal response indicates that rebalancing has occurred.

Perhaps you will inquire as to why this works. Answers will come if the question is engaged while the event is happening.

REBALANCING AT THE CRANIOVERTEBRAL JUNCTION

Our work at the craniovertebral junction will include evaluation of the major muscles involved in securing the head and upper neck in a network of muscular function, vestibular function, posture, and the horizontal orientation of the eyes, which connects elements in the neurological pathway known as the oculo-vestibular-cephalic function.

All muscles in the craniovertebral junction emerge from a center point and function as a unit. This represents Osteopathic thinking based on embryological research. The circle functions as a single muscle. All movements of the head and eyes around the circle are also passed to the vestibular mechanism, where balance is adjusted to the postural movements in the whole body.

The beauty of all this is further realized when one reflects on the center point. This is the seed from which all the muscles (the whole circle) sprouted. As growth occurs, the circle gets bigger and the muscles move further apart. The muscles act as one syncytium unless damaged.

In hyperextension injuries to these muscles (whiplash), a desynchronization of the wholeness of the circle is possible. Usually there are injuries to specific muscles that weaken in their capacity to move within the whole. The result is residual light-headedness, disequilibrium, headache, or even vertigo. Muscle-testing these small muscles can be done using eye movements or difficult voluntary micro-movements by the patient. Once a muscle weakness is noted, restoration of function can be accomplished by excitation of the antagonist muscle. Treatment response is almost immediate.

For rebalancing, go to the center point, find the connection to the Sea Around Us, and wait…

REBALANCING THE WHOLE FLUID BODY

The Fluid Body needs to be checked at the end of each treatment that promotes the engagement of Primary Respiration as a therapeutic force.

Checking for the need for rebalancing was encouraged by Dr. Sutherland as an act of safety. Dr. Wales, even after fifty years of practice, would routinely rebalance patients.

Briefly:

1) Check the Fluid Body for un-physiological motions of any kind. Normal would be a Fluid Body breathing as a single unit with only one fulcrum around which the whole moves or stills.
2) If you need to rebalance, appreciate the central stillness of the fulcrum (bigger than the fulcrum) and let your attention rest.
3) Wait without focusing on resolution.
4) When the Fluid Body breathes with the same rate and amplitude for three cycles, the treatment is over.

BALANCED MEMBRANOUS TENSION

As one who has been around Osteopathy in the cranial field since 1966, I have to say that I have heard many lectures on balanced membranous tension (BMT).

Most of them were dissimilar. There were considerable variations from the elders, and the descriptions in *Contributions of Thought* were quite wonderful but easily misinterpreted, unless one remembered that a lesion is *named and engaged through "what it can do."* That is its Direction of Ease.

All the methods you have heard and perhaps use are valid and probably safe ... but do they take the part into the whole? One must think about this question for a long time because the whole is creating the part and its location.

My history goes back to 1966 and the years between here and there. As I studied, I met several wonderful people who had studied with Sutherland from the early 1930s to his death. These people were part of his personal study group. They studied and taught with him his whole career. I was mentored for many years by Anne Wales, Ruby Day, and Rollin Becker, and for three years by George Laughlin, Dr. Still's grandson. All of these persons treated as if they were not "adding force" to the relationship with the lesion. They were quiet for long periods during treatment while they *listened* to the "Mechanism," a term used to describe a wholeness that was both inside and outside of the patient.

As they trained me, I eventually taught a lot of courses with the Sutherland Cranial Teaching Foundation (SCTF) and formed study groups that still function today. At each SCTF course I attended (25+), the explanation of BMT was slightly but importantly different.

Some practitioners disengaged the articulation and then went in the

Direction of Ease and into barrier with a varying amount of force, and waited for a therapeutic event. Most commonly witnessed was "tissue creep," or a release of the tension in the lesion makeup. In a sense one could say these were direct action methods because the Direction of Ease was minimized by two things, holding and barrier. All this was interesting and confusing, because interviews with Sutherland stated that he preferred the indirect method. So there was a dilemma in the air.

Years passed ... Around 1982 I asked Anne Wales why there was so much variation ... The answer was a huge surprise!

She stated clearly that Sutherland found it difficult to teach BMT because Osteopaths wanted to move the bones and BMT was about the membrane or the envelope around the tissue ... She said, and I repeat, there is no sense of bony tissue when one does BMT ... I felt caught in a truth I had never explored, even after nearly 30,000 cranial treatments ... I was sure I was listening and interacting with bone ... I was dumbfounded. She proceeded to teach me what Sutherland had taught her.

First let's revisit anatomy Osteopathically, as Still saw it. Osteopathic anatomy is based on the activity of involuntary motion in a dynamic ever-changing landscape very different from a picture in gross anatomy texts. We must make our anatomy alive and truly scientific while being open to what we honestly do not know...! What we do not know is very great. Using limited knowledge as some kind of absolute is a mistake. There are no authorities in any branch of science. Keep watching for what you never saw before and you will be doing what Still and Sutherland spent long hours doing. This kind of attitude and effort is very humbling, rewarding, and exciting.

THE JOURNEY FROM BARRIERS TO MOTION PRESENT

Language Can Be a Problem in This Profession

The terms "balanced ligamentous tension" (BLT) and "balanced membranous tension" (BMT) can be confusing if you study with a variety of teachers. The variations that have crept into the "original techniques" are all valid, but students are often confused as to what is correct technique ... everyone is correct. What is missing is an accurate description of what modifications an individual teacher might prefer to teach.

This commentary is about the history of what preceded Biodynamics in the work of Dr. Sutherland.

The principles of Osteopathy in the cranial field are designed to cooperate with Primary Respiration, with the Tide, but this is not all that Sutherland's teaching contained. He also taught work on the extremities and thorax that he acquired from Dr. Still that did not engage Primary Respiration, called balanced ligamentous tension, or BLT. In *Contributions of Thought*, Sutherland reports directly of Still's teaching:

> In technic we endeavor to follow Dr. Still's methods. That is, getting to the point of release with no jerking and then allowing the natural agencies to return the bones to their normal relations and positions. What are the natural agencies? The ligaments, not the muscles, are the natural agencies for this purpose of correcting the relations and positions at the joints.
> "Dr. Still's application of the technic is the gentle exaggeration

of the lesion that allows the natural agencies to draw the bones into place. Dr. Still has taken my hand in his and allowed me to feel the lesion as it was being exaggerated (the Direction of Ease), and then the natural agencies pulled the bones back into place. There is reason for applying that technic in the cranial mechanism. The difference between spinal technic and cranial technic is like the difference between an automobile mechanic and a watchmaker.

"We do not force anything into place in the reduction of a lesion. We have direction of the normal. (*Contributions of Thought*, 1944).

What Is Dr. Still Doing in His Demonstration to Dr. Sutherland?

He is taking the lesion in the Direction of Ease. We find the lesion field by its inertia, but we use the motion to treat ... This motion is gently increased (exaggerated) along the direction of least resistance, i.e., the Direction of Ease. At a point of balance or Neutral, the ligaments begin to move the bones.

From Sutherland's commentaries we find that he rarely recommends trying to reduce tissue tensions directly by manipulating the restriction into a release. A great discussion of this is in A Manual of Cranial Technique by the Lippincotts.

Consider how you treat. Do you use the Direction of Ease or do you encounter resistance under your hands as you treat? If you do, then there are some new horizons for you to explore if you wish to "feel and think" like Drs. Still and Sutherland.

The motion in the lesion is connected to the Health. As one matures, the thread that connects these two motions becomes evident.

The thread gives direction and power in the healing process. Without this particular skill it is not possible to engage Primary Respiration as a healing force, period.

BLT in its conception was a variety of principles, which are in the 1949 Academy of Applied Osteopathy Yearbook ... if you wish the true background story, study this writing. There are many modified teachings, which are good, but knowing the history creates an understanding of many things that may otherwise escape you. Learning BMT is not enough; one must know how to think from the forces behind the outcome ... and sense their activity in the process of resolution.

The principles of balanced ligamentous tension depend on the central nervous system and the spinal cord to do the work, to de-facilitate the segments and produce a change in ligamentous tensions that cause the bony position to move to a more natural location. The agencies creating the treatment are the physician's force and the neural network in the spinal cord that monitors the ligaments, not Primary Respiration. There are a variety of methods. I will discuss some, but I recommend that you write to the American Academy of Osteopathy and request the Academy of Applied Osteopathy Yearbook 1949, and read the section entitled "The Osteopathic Technique of William G. Sutherland, D.O.," by Howard Lippincott, D.O. ... This text covers the principles of Still as given to Sutherland and has photos of Will treating. This will be enlightening and historically accurate. It is the foundation of the language and ideas that led to the later work in the cranium called balanced membranous tension.

Balanced ligamentous tension is the prototype for balanced membranous tension involving the same principles using the membranes of the cranium (dura mater) ... the word "membrane" was taken from the word *meninges*... so the membrane called dura mater was originally seen as a ligament that could be used as an agency for correction of cranial bone lesions, replicating the model called Balanced Ligamentous Tension used on the peripheral segments. Sutherland refocused the cause behind the treatment to Primary Respiration, rather than using physician forces and the spinal reflex pathways to release the inertia ... What he discovered was that the lesion would transmute under the influence of the Tide ... This took many hard years to see into, but he kept asking, "Where is the fulcrum?" and "Where is the cause behind the treatment?"

Today, we endeavor to follow this thread that took Sutherland through a series of milestones, each one demanding a new way of being and thinking ... we ourselves will find the task to be full, demanding, and fulfilling.

BALANCED MEMBRANOUS TENSION

BMT Style #1

Motion test.

Find the pattern of resistance in the lesion field, and match it (mold to it).

Hold onto the barrier at the interface between your force and the inertia of the resistance in the tissue. Wait ...

Tissue creeps, moves involuntarily toward a balance point with less tension ... the therapeutic agency is the central nervous system, not Primary Respiration ... no transmutation occurs. This influences only the tensions matched, not the whole patient directly. We will not use this model.

BMT Style #2

Disengage the joint space.

Motion test.

Identify the permitted motion.

Go in the Direction of Ease.

Go past ease, slightly into barrier.

Wait for a release.

The end point is when the tissue releases.

Patient cooperation and/or thoracic respiratory cooperation are often added. We will not use this method.

BMT Style #3

Motion test and go in the Direction of Ease.

Continue following ease ...

The tissue melts (transmutes) into fluid.

Follow the fluid in the direction of its ease until it is still (reaches a balance point that matches the air in the room).

Wait for Thoracic Respiration to enter the balance point (Neutral). The Neutral is affected by Thoracic Respiration and the treatment spreads to the whole patient.

THE SUTURES

The theory that Sutherland first proposed about cranial motion was that the dural tissue acted like a ligament and moved the cranial base. From this cause the remaining bones, including the sacrum, were moved by mechanical forces translated from the center to the periphery.

In the cranium, the motion traveled from the base to the face and the vault, through the motion of mechanical gears. The gearing was along the sutures, which had unique shapes to accomplish three-dimensional motion in the whole head secondary to "gearing."

The sacrum was theoretically moved by dural tissue that extended from the head to the sacrum; this was called the "core-link."

Additionally, the dural motion was thought to cause the fluctuation of the cerebrospinal fluid, which caused the cranial rhythmic impulse. In a conversation with Anne Wales in 1953, Dr. Sutherland said he did not know what was moving the cranium. He apparently left the old model behind … a courageous act, for a lot was at stake. But this was a good lesson for us about humility.

Over recent years, our study of the cranium during its slower rates has allowed us to "see" the cranium in "slow motion," helping us to understand cranial motion in the head and sacrum in a different light, one that helps explain the whole and also leaves the theory open to change as we mature.

One of the principles we see in the metabolic motion in embryos and adults is that space opens and function moves into that space as the same form as the shape that was imprinted by a mysterious epigenetic force in the neutral protoplasm … we call this Primary Respiration, and the embryologists call it biodynamic forces.

Space opens and function moves in. The Direction of Ease.

What many of us "see" is the sutures opening in the first stages of breathing and the bones changing shape, breathing, into the space created. Let's take a look at how the abrogation of the central nervous system occurs in an embryo to learn more about this idea.

Early in the development of the central nervous system, before there is any cortex, the future cortex cells are clustered around the outside of the third ventricle. Outside of this there are empty fluid fields. Before cells move from the outer wall of V3 to the periphery and become cortex, a strange and beautiful event occurs. Inside the empty fluid appears a shape, like a tree. This shape opens and the future cortex cells "drift" in the motion of the whole into the space of the shape of the tree. This arborization creates canals where the cells can make passage easily toward their destinations. The space opens, then the function moves in. This is worth reading about, as the story is very Osteopathic and helpful.

In our infancy, early in this program, we proposed that the embryological forces were present throughout life and accounted for the odd things we observe in the fluids in adults. This theory has proven quite useful and in fact some embryologists and neurophysiologists are beginning to have the same idea ... but there is as yet little interest in the theory because the practical use of the hands as tools has not been forthcoming. However, Still definitely saw the innate healing forces as a continuum from birth, not separate from growth and development.

Our theory has played out very well in practice.

You may think it is obvious. The training many of us had from 1965 to 1978 made this physiological understanding a challenge. Now the idea is very popular but not necessarily as a part of Thinking Osteopathy. Sometimes truth ends up as words, not relationship.

Ideas are not for power but for humility ... what we know ever more and more is how little we know. This sets the stage for a "new beginning" on a regular basis. What we know must be left behind during treatment so we can see more and more of the laws essential to health … laws not made up by the human intellect, but by expression of the Creator.

Therefore, the Mystery cannot end, and in that insecurity is freedom from the slavery of the past and a pause where something enters the space and shapes the mind. There is a filling up of space with something "new", and the old ends.

HEALING AND THE NATURAL WORLD

In January 1997, the interview "Jim Jealous, DO Healing and the Natural World" appeared in *Alternative Therapies in Health and Medicine,* Vol 3, No. 1.

It is reprinted here with kind permission from the copyright holder InnoVision Professional Media.

CONVERSATIONS

JIM JEALOUS, DO
HEALING AND THE NATURAL WORLD

Interview by Bonnie Horrigan • Photography by Dan Higgins

There is a reason that people drive from neighboring states to see Jim Jealous, DO, at his clinic in Vermont. It is the same reason that students line up to take his classes and that the University of New England College of Osteopathic Medicine founded a scholarship in his name—the James Jealous Scholarship for Excellence in Osteopathic Medicine. Dr Jealous has dedicated his life to exploring the natural world in its most essential, fundamental form and it is this knowledge and the resultant skill that makes him one of the most respected osteopathic doctors in America today.

Dr Jealous graduated from the Kirksville College of Osteopathy and Surgery in 1970 and is certified by the American Osteopathic Board at special proficiency in osteopathic and manipulative medicine. In private practice since 1971, he runs a clinic in Milton, Vermont and is a clinical instructor at the University of New England College of Osteopathic Medicine. Dr Jealous, a member of American Academy of Osteopathy, the American Osteopathic Association, and the Cranial Academy, is past president of the Osteopathic Center for Children in London and a prior member of the Sutherland Cranial Teaching Foundation.

Alternative Therapies *interviewed Dr Jealous at his clinic in Milton Vermont in the fall of 1996.*

Alternative Therapies: Our philosophy is that while conventional medicine is very effective in many situations, it doesn't have all the answers. That's what I'd like to talk to you about—the answers conventional medicine doesn't have.

James Jealous: Let's look at the conditions in medical education. The whole process of becoming a physician is largely contradictory to the principles of healing. Students are not nurtured, nor are they encouraged to explore, nor are they communicated with as fellow travelers in a remarkably beautiful journey into the mountains of life. The healing arts have become quite sterile and the biomolecular view of healing has distinct limits, limits that trim off the "individual." This, of course, is a reflection of the educational ecosystem. The growth and development of a physician should be nurtured by the most loving and perceptive environment that is humanly possible. This is paramount to bring a complete picture of illness into focus.

Osteopathy in its conception contained a philosophy as well as a science. Osteopaths were asked to consider questions of the soul, death, transcendence, and use only their hands in healing. The background in which life occurs has meaning. I believe that any healing art needs to help individuals find the way to a deeper reality than a biomolecular model of health.

It is interesting to me to see how many alternative medical models are slowly becoming biomolecular. Many "natural" cures are really biomolecular remedies and are used like traditional medicine uses "drugs." From my perception that's not necessarily alternative, because an alternative medical practice would be of a larger vision and be very individualized in its application. It would not have a remedy for each symptom or disease, but a unique option for the patient. The deeper questions about life need to enter into the picture and be part of the inquiry about healing. We are oversimplifying the art and losing the essence of what healing is about. Holistic is not using a variety of "cures," it is seeing the Spirit, Soul, Body as a Whole. The treatment is not subdivided; if it is, then one must see one's position relative to the Whole and not try and "destroy the disease" (allopathic) but support the health of the Whole. This was osteopathy's beginning; it remains barely alive, but is practiced by several hundred DOs.

The idea of Whole, a unit, the undivided, is foreign to our culture and is slowly vanishing like an aboriginal form that is viewed as "primitive" by the intellect. Each one of us faces the reality in ourselves and must meet that responsibility first, then the perception will follow. For our culture it's a "deep" question; for the aboriginal soul it's a natural state. We need to focus not so much on cause and effect but on the priority of the Whole as it moves in relation to a Great Mystery. Teaching requires an effort in the same direction, a view of the Whole individual moving into new dimensions of life. We need to protect the eco-receptive perception that is our natural state of being. This is slowly being trimmed away and as a result, people are more sick than necessary. If they become ill, their inner balance and "peace of mind" are not juxtaposed to the causal event, and as a result, suffering is increased. The same process is present during education.

Reprint requests: InnoVision Communications, 101 Columbia, Aliso Viejo, CA 92656. Tel, (800) 899-1712 or (714) 362-2050 (ext 532); fax, (714) 362-2022; e-mail, ivcReprint@aol.com.

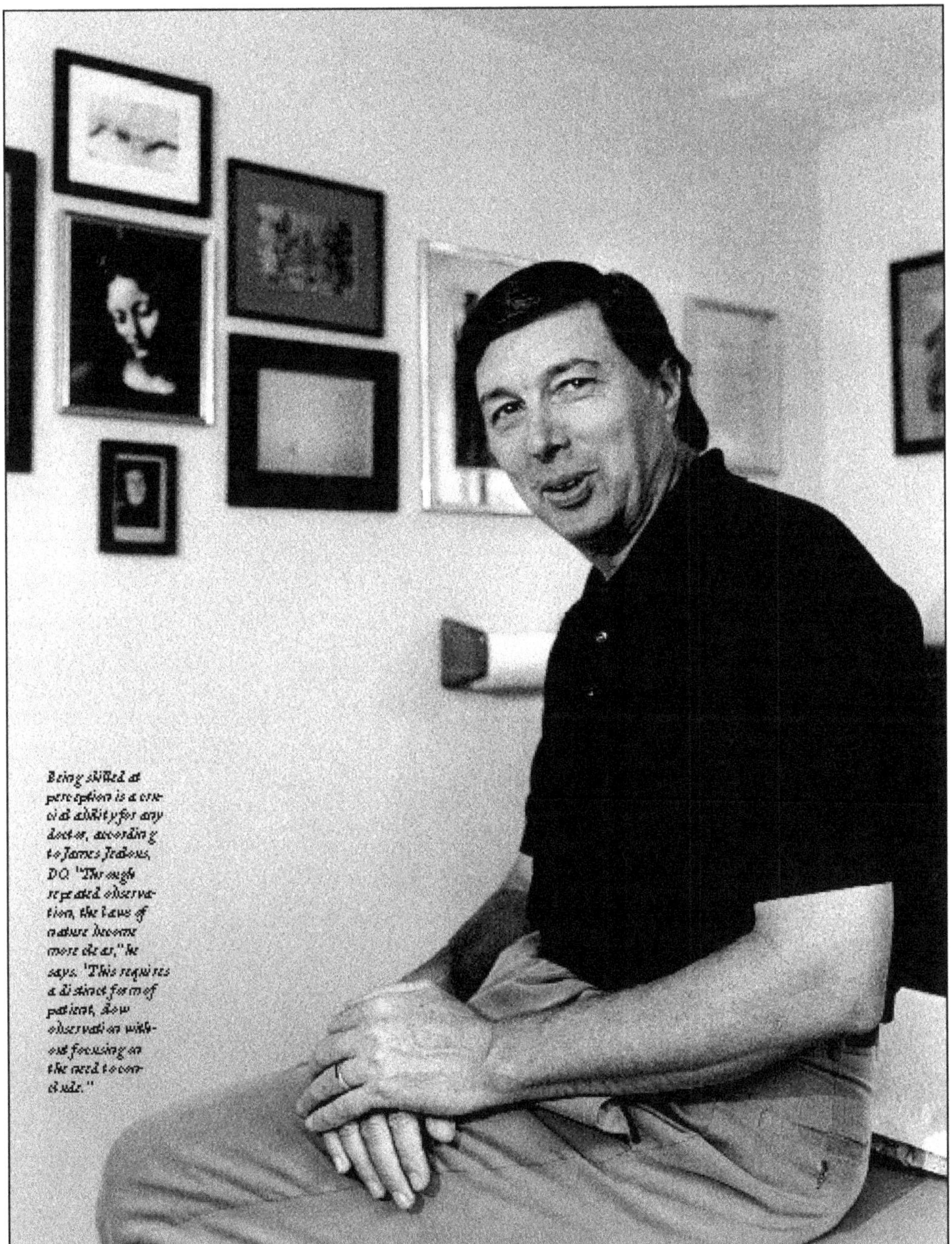

Being skilled at perception is a crucial ability for any doctor, according to James Jealous, DO. "Through repeated observation, the laws of nature become more clear," he says. "This requires a distinct form of patient, slow observation without focusing on the need to conclude."

If we are seeking an alternative system of healthcare, then training must reflect that difference. Philosophy is not enough. We must try and live the principles. Physicians must not prioritize their relationship with the patient around time. This is a serious problem. An office call for an acute illness requires at least a half hour.

AT: Not 7 minutes?

Jealous: I'm not bright enough to practice medicine in 7 minutes. Taking longer is necessary and prudent, but also it's economical. I mention this because alternative medicine should not be more expensive. An osteopathic treatment is usually applied once (for an acute illness), the patient has a perception on why they got ill and how that impacts their essential goals in life, and recovers more quickly without medications. Long-term patients begin to "manage" their inner balance and learn about staying healthy. All this requires remarkably less healthcare. Healers are teachers, fellow travelers, and explorers. Patients are in similar roles within the sphere of their lives. We are here to free people from needing routine healthcare, not create dependence. Short, quick office calls leave the patient frustrated and dependent; they either keep coming or break away and find their own way. The medical care in the United States is trying to "herd" people like cows. People are essentially spirited and will find their way forward on their own. Routine healthcare is becoming less and less sensitive. Interesting.

AT: Is this type of thinking the foundation of osteopathic medicine?

Jealous: At the foundation, yes, but is it the status quo? No. Like all schools of healing, the deeply essential core is the least evident. The individual is still the key answer; we can't blame who we are on anything. Some people just desire to serve as much as possible the Health in each of us; not fight diseases. Most DOs have bought into the status, materiality, and fear of the mainstream medical model. The exceptions that we find prove the potential of our philosophy. Only a small number of DOs continue to explore our foundations.

AT: What are those foundations?

Jealous: Our aim is to learn about the natural laws using the perceptual skills that we develop in our training and practice. The core of this work is perceptual; the concept grew out of repeated observation until the laws of nature became more clear. We learn to sense the Whole. When one meets a patient one sees the Whole—a very unique and rare event in our modern world. One does not divide life into soma/psyche/visceral, etc. This is an event contained only in the moment one is in. It's extra-ordinary. Patients are very much aware that a different attention is present. They comment on it. It's not intellectual or intuitive. It's aboriginal, instinctual. There is no immediate conclusion or diagnosis—that's much later. The moment is filled with the effort to be present with the Health in the patient and the story as it unfolds into its own answer. Sometimes this requires a distinct form of patient, slow observation without focusing on a need to conclude. The process is foreign at first, but after a time one finds it quite natural as it essentially is. We learn our skills by apprenticeship to something that has no name but it teaches us a great deal. We learn sensory perception without conceptual overlay, but it runs deeper than one can imagine. Learning this is different and demanding. Very few people are dedicated to this form of living; their interests are otherwise. So our profession is largely allopathic, and that's a loss for everyone.

We use our hands diagnostically, perceptually, and therapeutically—that's how simple and profound this is. We are not listening for symptoms but for a pre-established priority set in motion by the Health in the patient. The founder of osteopathy, an MD surgeon, had a vision and followed his insight. He trained physicians to use their hands for healing, along with very simple and natural remedies—diet, rest, meditation, prayer—nothing was added but "hands-on healing." It works!

AT: Talk more about natural laws.

Jealous: Well, first of all they are not man-made. Not conceived by research other than observation. Secondarily, we are aware that many laws exist and operate in healing that we are completely unaware of, and yet they still enter profoundly into the process. The interesting thing is that our perception can sense the intention of natural laws, the intention of the Health at work, where priorities are being established. Usually, once this is communicated, the patient is already aware of it but may have discarded the information. Our motive and our skill is to understand the intention of the Health in the patient as it works undivided in pursuing balance and harmony. As I said earlier, this is not limited by terminal disease.

After being trained to sense this reality in a hands-on practice one feels very blessed to be an osteopath. Many people don't sense the beauty of this and use a more mechanical model and align structure to improve health by removing neuromuscular barriers. This is fine work but not of a continued interest for many DOs.

The natural world is endowed with a consciousness that extends in all directions. Our numbers are limited by time, interest, and teachers. It takes years, and then some, it's a way of life, really. My idea of alternative medicine is an alternative perception of the world, not just disease. Osteopathy has been alternative since 1874. We are still here. Alternative medicine, to me, is about a different view of life, a more reverent and deeply informative beauty. Giving tea tree oil for nail fungus instead of a potentially toxic chemical is a much more natural remedy, but it's still not an alternative view of healing. Any form or "mindset" that goes after the disease to override it is only partially alternative. What supports the Whole at its interface with the wisdom of the natural world is alternative. It supports the Health, the non-divisible, the transcendent wisdom of life, first. In ordinary illness, rarely is more required. About 80% of all common illnesses will heal with this approach, if the patient is past postgraduate.) It's heart-to-hands. The hardest lesson to teach is to work at the tempo of the Health. We don't hack away at disease. You know, 3 minutes of waiting is torture for some people. We need time, "free" time.

Students learn that they already are "skilled," perceptive. We allow what is natural to emerge; they surprise themselves. Very few teachers try and help us see the dynamic life we are. We don't need to become enlightened, we are. We need to sense our wholeness, we relax into this beauty and begin. Life by itself is beautiful. I'm not blinded by the violence and suffering. I see it and I see something "other" sustaining us. In medicine this focus is missing. My experience with mainstream medicine is not a pleasant one because of its focus. Fifteen or so years ago I had a swelling in my thyroid. I saw several specialists and was told that I had cancer. They were all very nervous, excitable, disturbed; they lacked insight and were afraid of my cancer. They laid out a morbid picture. I was very scared. I told them I was not coming back, because I realized from their fears that I was afraid of dying. It surprised me because I thought I loved life enough to die without fear. I decided that I needed to come to peace with death and not work out of fear. The doctors were angry. I never told anyone. I just decided that I wanted to be free of the fear. It was a question of integrity with the gift of living.

I did not touch the growth for one and a half years. I did this because it really was frightening to feel it and think about death, cancer, and a "void." I worked at not letting myself forget how afraid I was of death. Then I'd go about my day. Nothing else. I really tried to see my fear and help it through this misunderstanding. It went away. The growth went away and it never returned. I'm not claiming a self cure. I have no idea what happened or why. But I had a choice between my spirit and fear. I am proud to be part of nature, I love nature. I am proud to be mixed in with the trees and the sun and everything. This feeling of wholeness was violated by the fear. I could not stop loving what gave me form and consciousness. I took my fear along with me and continued. We are enlightened, we know we belong intimately to life, and it's precious, it keeps giving each of us 100% without reservation. It's simply true.

AT: Does osteopathy have a definition for death?

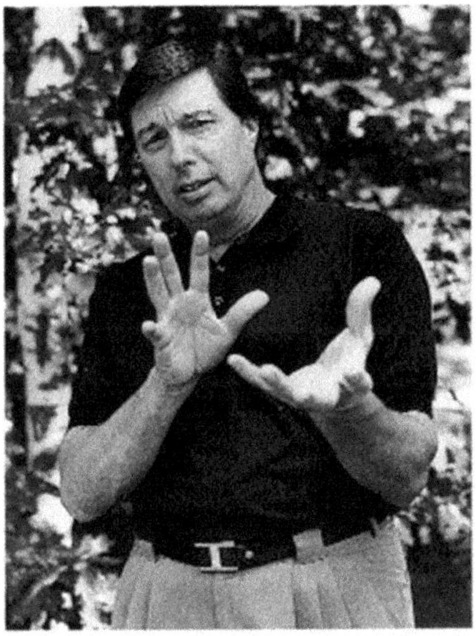

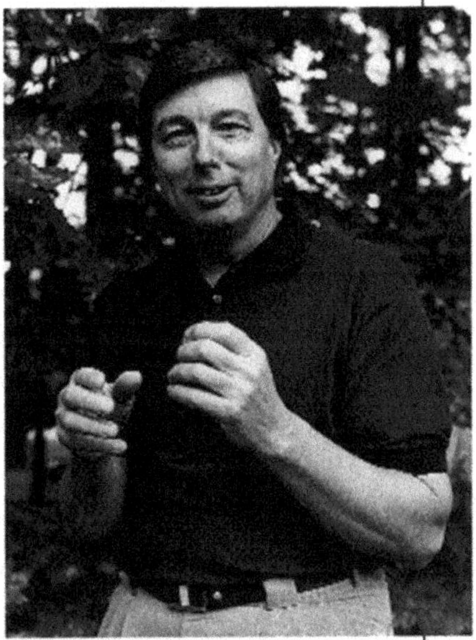

Jealous: The founder, AT Still, MD, said, "The body is a second placenta." I guess the question is best answered by saying death does not exist. I don't superimpose my understanding on the patient. I support all their decisions once they are clear about their choice of healthcare. I have patients from all sides of the issues. My job is to remain aware of the "undiseasable" health in them and support it. Patients are skilled; it takes humility to come for help. When I place my hands on a patient I begin by sensing the wholeness, the transcendent, not as an idea or as an immortal truth but by waiting until it is evident. I see the fear, I feel it in my hands, I sense the disease, the lesions, the history, and I wait. I'm looking for what I don't know; not a diagnosis, that's later. Now in this moment the Health is interfacing with disease. This priority must be seen directly, not by deduction.

AT: How would you change our healthcare system to accommodate this?

Jealous: If we look at whether or not we can change the healthcare system in this country, we can't. We want things to change because we believe differently than other people, but certainly people who practice medicine have a right to practice medicine their way, and there are patients who prefer different formats. I don't think it's our place to dictate what should be done.

We've never had a safe, intelligent, and effective haven for people who want to practice holistic medicine. We need to acknowledge them. Instead of putting them down because they want to spend time with the patients, we need to say, "That's fine." There needs to be some form of recognition. I don't think we're

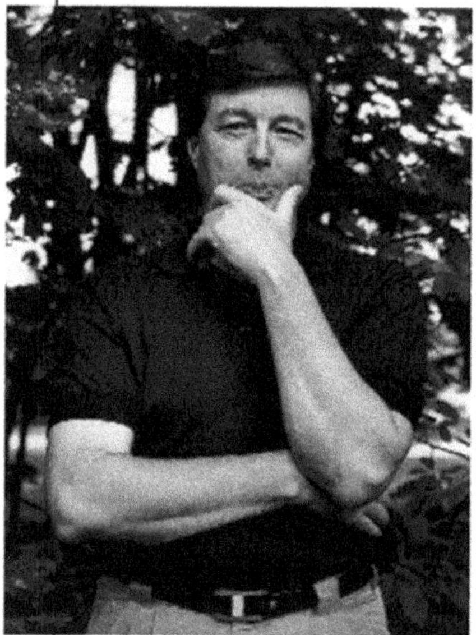

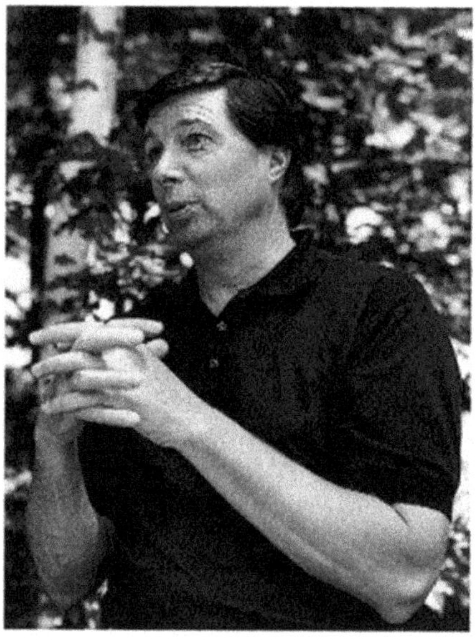

that the cause of the origin of the embryo is held within the consciousness of the embryo itself. That's not a direct quote, but there was a secret, a mystery, that must remain. One can sense it's genesis. It is at the center of the Healing process.

Blechschmidt was fascinated by the fact that there was a force inside the fluids of the body that was not coming from the genetic field. This force inside the fluid actually contains the idea of the form of the human body, whether it's a kidney or vertebra or eye, and it brings it into manifestation. Then the genes modify it. So we have genetic/cultural and race modifications. Before these modifications, there is divine form. It coexists during our whole life. There is a moment when we're all perfectly held in the matrix of a much finer Intention, a moment of healing.

going to change the healthcare system in this country, because it's not being run by physicians. The psyche, the metaphoric content, behind the healthcare system is the same thing that's happening in the movies and everything else. It's fast food. People want action and they want it right now.

Maybe I'm ignorant, but I think it's foolish to try to change anything by dictation. What makes alternative medicine what it is, if it's going to be anything, are the individuals. Instead of having everybody recruiting other people, I'd rather see them in their offices, working. Let students come to them. Make them work. Because it is work. Stand on the center and wait.

AT: Let's go back to the subject of healing.

Jealous: Healing is the emergence of originality. Let's take a look at this one sentence for a moment. The breath of life comes into the body. We can sense various rhythms that are created from it, and we can perceive that process taking place. We're not interpolating it. We're not analyzing it. We can actually perceive the breath of life come into the body, come to the midline, and from the midline, generate different forms of rhythms in the bioelectric field, fluids, and tissue. Essentially, what's happening is genesis. It never stops. Moment to moment we are building new form and function. One senses this, directly.

When I was reading the embryology literature, [I found the] research done by a German man named Blechschmidt. He was a scientist in love with embryos. His question was about the biodynamics and biokinetics of human development. How does this thing work? What happens? He never got his answer. He wrote

Blechschmidt described six different ways in which fluids will interact with each other inside the body. William Sutherland, who is the founder and genius of osteopathy in the cranial field, perceived these forces in the fluids, yet the two men had never met or read each other's work. When I read that this embryologist was describing the same forces in the fluids as one of the great teachers of osteopathy, that's all it took.

Since then, I've spent a lot of time just looking at pictures of embryos in the first 6 weeks of life, before the genetic field takes over. Many people won't agree with what I'm saying, or perhaps they will misinterpret it, but these forces exist. Many old cultures recognize this truth. But how did they know it? They knew it because it was something they perceived, directly, a natural occurrence.

Now, are we just taking a philosophical trip or is there some practical knowledge in the perception and understanding that there's a force breathing into the body 24 hours a day? It's on watch, it's on call, working for the patient. It cannot become diseased. It's before that. All it does is carry the original form into that person. And it's the thing that emerged from the man that had cancer when he knew he was dying. It's what we would call "his spirit." Why it came the way it came in that moment in time, we don't know. But it interfaces with every moment of our life. The air pollution coming in our nose, the good thoughts we have, our hair, our age, how much we have to urinate. It interfaces with every moment and if it stopped being there, you wouldn't die, you'd dissolve. You would have no matrix for your consciousness, even after death.

Let's say, 3 years ago, you hit your head, and ever since you've had dizziness. You've had all kinds of medicine, and nothing worked. You've still got the vertigo. If you walked into my office and I put my hands on you, I would not be looking for the strain pattern in your body. I wouldn't look at your disease. I observe the breath of life, this force in the body that's unchangeable, and look at how it was trying to help you. Your illness was precognitive. It knew you were going to walk into that wall before you did, not in a psychological way, but perceptually, something knew.

AT: Are you talking about premonitions?

Jealous: I'm not talking about premonitions. If you talk to enough people who have automobile accidents, just milliseconds before it happens, they know it. I'm talking about how the body is set up to receive the shock, whether it was emotional, biochemical, genetic, or physical. So the treatment program is set up almost before, and certainly during, the process of the insult to the body, or spirit, or soul.

The blueprint to get the patient well is there because the thing that made the body is the thing that sets up the blueprint. It creates compensation, to hold balance—what we call homeostasis—as long as possible. Now I know that a physician hearing this would say, "This is crazy." Some ideas of health are extremely narrow-minded, so death is an insult to a physician. But it's much bigger than that. We can feel the movement of this force inside the body, unchanged in the adult from that of a newborn, and for 2 or 3 days after death. Then it seems to disappear. Now, I won't go into that, because that's getting on the edge and there are a lot of things I don't know about it. But I think Elizabeth Kübler-Ross has done a great service for humanity. She made us wake up to the fact that there was more to life than just what was apparent to us. She put love on the front line. It wasn't emotional love. It was an unconscious awareness of a bond that exists between every human being before you even meet the person. It's very much a reality.

AT: Tell me more about the practice of osteopathy.

Jealous: The patient comes into the office. He's banged his head, he's got the vertigo. It's been going on for 3 years. So if we put our hands on the patient's body, the first thing we do is we open our senses to the peripheral space in the room, and extend it to the horizon, by its own force. Not by intention. A lot of people like to use their intention, their attention, and they like to visualize. I know enough anatomy to know that if I tried to visualize anatomy, I would be making a terrible mistake, because there's so much variability. For me, those elements of intention, attention, and visualization don't enter into this therapeutic process. They have places in other motifs but not in this.

Just like your lungs breathe in and out, attention breathes in and out. You know how you can relax the abdomen so you're not breathing up top all the time? What would happen if your mind was allowed to breathe?

Instead of working with breath, or air, we work with the breath of life. We let the mind breathe. This takes hard work. Some people start crying after they do it for the first time because they realize they were handmade, on purpose, by an artist who loves his work. They feel completely embraced by life and they get the magic. Then one struggles to get it to come back. That's when they fail because you have to let go of it. The first step in feeling this breath of life is not about palpation or poking around looking for lesions. You're feeling the Health of the patient first. You're feeling the breath of life as it comes into that living organism, into that person, and you're feeling the body, soul, and spirit as a complete unit of function. One does not partition. If you divide the body, soul, and spirit, even conceptually, under your hands, you're not doing what I'm talking about. You're doing something else.

I'm not talking about putting your hands on a person and saying, "This person is nervous," or he's having a bad day. That's intuition. This is a totally different thing. You feel the breath of life come into the body and up the midline. The midline is a bioelectric line that's a remnant of the notochord formed in the embryonic plate. It's a primary line of orientation for all spatial dynamics. The breath of life comes in along that line, and then it creates changes in the body. It creates movements, fluids, tissues, and so forth. We feel that.

This Health in the patient has been trying to heal him since the disease was imprinted. So in the case of the person with the vertigo, the Health has been working on it for 3 years. It has the blueprint to heal it. Now, the most common question I get right now from students is, "Why doesn't it heal the patient without our help?"

AT: I was just about to ask you that.

Jealous: When you get into the vortex of the interface between the healing forces and distortion, there could be 100 pounds per square inch of pressure being held in the distortion. The force of the insult set up vectors in the body. I don't wish this on anyone, but let's say you saw a friend run over by an automobile. How many pounds per square inch do you think that shock is putting into your system? A lot. Enough so you could lift an automobile off the ground if you had to. Let's suppose that this healing force could balance out that hundred pounds per square inch in your body. If you put a hundred pounds per square inch of force into the body, you would rupture every artery, vein, and lymphatic. If it generated the force necessary to heal it directly, its own architecture would collapse.

So there's no gain. In other words, it has to heal through transubstantiation, which is changing the physical force into another form of force that it can deal with. At a certain point of softening, very quickly, just like the snap of a finger, it switches into another form of energy. The information for that change is coming from the breath of life. So the disproportion of the lesion or injury or disease is bounded on all sides. The disease process is an intelligent decision made by the breath of life to protect the organism from destroying the whole of itself. Disease is not the enemy. It's an intelligent, wise decision to come into balance.

Think about death. What do you reclaim at death?

AT: Your original form.

Jealous: Right. Your original form. It's incredible when you see it. Do you know how many times, after a couple of treatments, a patient will say, "I feel more like myself." They will say, "I can see light moving across the surface of the leaves after it rains." I say, "It's always been there. That's not a mystical perceptual field. It's normal." We are naturally quite gifted.

What would happen if you claimed your original form? Wouldn't it be interesting to know who you were? Wouldn't it be interesting to know the intention of the breath of life when it made you?

AT: Do you talk about these types of things with your patients?

Jealous: This conversation I'm having with you, on a less detailed level, goes on with my patients most of the time. I'm not trying to talk them into it. I can't say I love them in the usual sense of the word, but I see something in them and I know it's coming out, and I ask, "Why not right now?"

Why don't they all get better? It's just not time. And that's the only answer. The patient should not be blamed for not getting well. If the standard medical people make mistakes in not giving patients enough time to understand the body, soul, and spirit as a unit, alternative healthcare practitioners make equally bad mistakes when they make the patient responsible for not being conscious enough to get well. It's no one's fault. It's more about tempo and "healing-time."

People aren't stupid. Most people are very bright. Some doctors think they're smarter than everybody else, but it's not true. We are all very human.

AT: How do you teach students to feel these forces?

Jealous: First, I tell them they can practice any way they want, as long as it's safe, effective, and intelligent. They may not choose to practice the way I do. So they watch me treat patients and I teach them based on their questions. Eventually, they want to imitate what I'm doing. So they imitate it a couple of times and it works, and they think they have it, and then it doesn't work any more. So they get self-critical, their self-confidence level drops.

I try to convince them that they are already completely skilled. I try to get them to uncover something extraordinary in themselves. It's just a matter of time. If they let their minds relax, and sit and listen to the patient the same way I do, they come up with answers. It usually takes about 2 years for them to accept this, before they'll try it with one patient. They may see seven, eight hundred patients on their own during that part of their training, but usually it's 2 years before they'll try it. Then they wait and begin to find the Health.

I received a letter from a student yesterday. I trained her for 5 years. She spent 400 hours intermittently with me before going into (a conventional) family practice residency. She was recently assigned to a 92-year-old woman who had been in good health until she developed a growth on her neck, which was a squamous-cell carcinoma.

My student wrote, "While [the patient's] physical condition quickly deteriorated, she was obviously fearful about what was happening to her, as was her family."

Now, here's an intern in a hospital, taking care of a terminally ill patient with a squamous-cell cancer. I think it's pretty good she noticed that the patient and her family are frightened. Anyway, to make a long story short, she wrote, "I found myself alone with the patient, which was a really rare moment. And while I was listening to her heart, I realized what I was really trying to do. On one level, I could feel the fear inside of this woman, almost a hum inside of her nervous system. But underneath it was a sweet, shapeless sense of certainty and health."

Then she wrote, "While I stayed there, I felt a huge shift." (She was treating the patient.)

Now that means that the partition between the fear and the sweetness let go. The autonomic nervous system, the parasympathetic, and sympathetics came more into balance, probably through the effect of the treatment on her limbic system. She felt a shift, which she couldn't describe. She then wrote, "The patient seemed to relax. She had a quiet, peaceful night, which was very unusual, and when I checked with her this morning, she seemed very comfortable. She died a few hours later."

An extraordinary story. We don't know, but there's a good possibility the treatment let her slip across easily. Did she hasten the process of death? No. She helped the patient come into balance, and then the system went in the direction it would naturally go. We didn't make that decision, and that's what makes osteopathy a natural science.

AT: There seems to be some magic in the moment when someone perceives the sweetness, the ineffable original force. That seems to be a key moment.

Jealous: It is a key moment. The recognition of the Health is a moment that's always there. You come to a conclusion about what the blueprint is and what it's trying to do, and you actually help it go in that direction. This may be a very subtle force.

You have to be right there at that interface, and you have to have watched and watched and watched it so that at that point where it interfaces, you can be present with the action of the blueprint.

AT: Is it like a little push?

Jealous: When you read the blueprint, you read the tone, the texture, the intention, the intensity, and the tempo as one thing. You've got all those five elements, plus. When they all balance, you accent exactly what is there.

There are other ways to treat that are effective, but we're talking specifically about the breath of life and its effect on the body.

AT: Any final words?

Jealous: I want to summarize the things I think are important.

First is that the whole is real. Holistic medicine doesn't mean that you do homeopathy, acupuncture, and osteopathy, and give them antibiotics. Holistic medicine means that the patient is indivisible. A person cannot be broken down. Holistic medicine means you have the ability to perceive the whole, and not partition it, which is a big responsibility.

We talked about the laws of generation and healing; healing as the emergence of originality, and that it can happen at any moment.

Another thing is perceptual training. You have to own the gift you are given. Sir Laurens Van der Post wrote some great books on perception. He is an extraordinary teacher. If you want to understand instinctual perception, his work with the aboriginals in Africa is a great resource.

In David Abrams' book, *The Spell of the Sensuous,* he talks to some medicine men who know about the six directions of perception. It's a good book to help a person explore reality. Three years ago I gave a lecture on perception, about the importance of the horizon in our perception. It was completely from my own experience. When I read Abrams' book, it was a good affirmation for me.

For me, the essence is to allow your attention to breathe over the edge of the horizon, set it free, and then wait for it to come back on its own. There's a perceptual bridge here that we can teach people.

The other thing that we talked about was that the treatment program for the patient is prioritized by the forces that form the body, so that when the patient comes in, the treatment program is already set up. We don't create the treatment process. We have to uncover it. That is a big sentence and it should be explored.

We talked about transmutation and about how death is not a disease.

It's important not to limit the patient to your practice. If you don't feel like you're helping the patient, get some help. If the patient doesn't want to go anywhere else, then find out why he's afraid. But keep expanding the influences on that patient's life, and don't hold on to the patient.

It's very interesting that the natural healing community has taken on the allopathic approach to medicine. The patient comes in with symptoms, and he gets symptom remedies. It's like prescribing prescription drugs. They're caught up in an intellectual format and they're not even aware of it. Natural medicine is natural medicine. Now, what does that word mean? Nature means everything that lives or breathes or is. So starlight? I bet a lot of people would get well if they just went for walks at night and could see the stars. All therapy is unique to the conditions of now, not the disease.

What good is it to start giving patients all kinds of things until we really understand what the whole process is? A real healer is not going to give exactly the same remedy for the same disease twice. So if we want to practice alternative medicine, we have to get rid of the menus. We have to look at the menus as a support system to buy time, but it's not the end of the road, and we are not all on the same timing.

Traditional osteopathy is not about episodic healthcare. It's a long-term relationship with people wherever you practice. It takes years to get to know another human being. Some of the people I've treated for 30 years. I'm not threatened by their disease, and I think that's important.

The other point that is important is that the student-teacher relationship is a long-term thing. We have to accept the responsibility of being taught. One of my greatest teachers was an old man I met on the river one day. I was way up country fishing and there was this incredible storm. He got in his car and headed back to town to his home. I didn't have anywhere else to go, so I asked him if I could come in his house. The storm came and his house trailer was rocking on its foundation. The electric wires were down in the road, and there were sparks all over the place. There were ambulances and cars coming from everywhere.

I sat there with this old man at the table, and he never moved. We just sat there. Inside this trailer was a hovering stillness. It was incredible. We were just sitting in this trailer with all this chaos going on. After 20 minutes, everything calmed down. He looked at me and said, "I never could understand why people would rush around to make an emergency out of life." Then he just sat there. Twenty minutes later, he got up and started cooking a meal. He knew how to let the moment be the source and center of his temple; he was a living reminder.

I subsequently became good friends with him. That was an important moment, because I realized that it's not just osteopaths who are doing this kind of work and who can understand what's happening in the moment or be awake to that breath of life and that stillness. We all are aware of something greater and need to remember our Originality.

The health maintenance organization that we're all looking for is what makes an embryo. It generates and maintains life.

I don't think there is anything wrong with centering your general practice on the whole human being. Not everybody is going to be interested, and not everybody is going to think that you're doing a great job. But that's not what it's about. What it's about is whether or not there's a general pattern to your practice that's useful to people and their well being.

And the last thing, in big black letters—it's hard work. So prepare to really live! Thank you.

BIODYNAMICS OF OSTEOPATHY BOOK SERIES

This book is one of a series of twelve *Biodynamics of Osteopathy* books. It is recommended that you read the whole series in order, as each book builds on the understanding from prior books. It is also recommended that you seek experienced teachers and mentors to help you experience the full depth of the information given.

The full series is as follows:

Phase One is about involuntary motion, which is motion present in the whole and in the lesion. We learn to synchronize with the breathing of Primary Respiration before we approach any treatment. This synchronization is the key to working with stable rates and not irritating the system. The principle of synchronizing with a healthy aspect of the patient suffuses the whole teaching program. This synchronization shifts our awareness to a different level of receptivity, which allows us to see Primary Respiration rather than the lesion field, and this eventually leads us to an understanding of the intention of Primary Respiration.

Phase Two is about communication with the natural laws of healing that surround activity at 2 to 3 cycles per minute. We synchronize with the breathing of Primary Respiration and also add the skill of sensing the fulcrum, the Stillness through which the breathing creates form and function. It is a different kind of synchronization from that in Phase One, shifting our awareness more deeply. As this occurs, the treatment automatically expresses itself. The end point of treatment, when compared with Phase One, reveals several differences. We find this kind of synchronization works exclusively with the fluid body and the outcome of treatment is more complete than when working with tissue alone.

Phase Three is centered around the activities of the Long Tide (100 second cycle). We explore an indwelling therapeutic force already present in the lesion field. We learn that the dural system is not made-up of three sickles but rather a series of folds in a sac, arising during growth and development. We see the relationship between the upper and lower dural sacs, awakening us to the independence of two separate tentorium cerebelli. We discover that zone D, the horizon, and the Wire (along which the Long Tide moves during its intended therapeutic course) are all linked as natural laws pertaining to this level of Primary Respiration.

Phase Four focuses on the Midline, a place where the spatial relationships are expressed as a whole. It synchronizes and centers us in such a way that we become aware of Zone D and the Dynamic Stillness. The Third Level Stillness in Phase Four is different from the Stillness in the other Phases – we are centered by the Stillness at the center of creation. Our intention is replaced by the intention of the Tide which can facilitate our spiritual path.

Phase Five is about *the face*. As we approach the face, we use all of the principles that we have learned in Phase One, Two, Three, and Four. We work with automatic shifting and notice differences from how the face is viewed by older models within Osteopathy in the Cranial Field. As we synchronize with the therapeutic presence of the Long Tide we see what we can learn about the face from that landscape. We also work with Seams, Dynamic Stillness, and Ignition.

Phase Six is a continuation of our journey into the Wholeness that generates life and delivers therapeutic forces that transmute lesions once Neutral is expressed. It is a mixture of activities centered around the outside presence of Primary Respiration as something that is a non-biological force and that has a persona. We will also continue to explore seams and then move on to the extremities, first in the embryological terms and then as Sutherland taught them in his work called PowerPoints. Phase 6 is a time to build your understanding of the Tide and refine your skills.

Phase Seven highlights the Health. Dr. Still's famous comment "Find the Health; anyone can find disease," has plagued many minds over the last century. We come to the clear vision of several indwelling aspects of the Health: Love … liquid light … and a diamond matrix. A approach to the terminally ill and dying patient is addressed. In the somatic sensation of the Tide passing through the House Under the Sea, our awareness is transmuted by the Health. The lesion is seen as a precognitive act of the Health. Thoracic Respiration, Primary Respiration, and Ignition are as One. The landscape is vast … and the principles of healing are even more substantial than we have previously experienced..

Phase Eight is a deeper exploration of seams, balanced rhythmic interchange, and the Flame of Intention as a therapeutic modality. Phase Eight is the culmination of our awareness of Wholeness, and ultimately brings us to the Divine Presence, Unconditional Love and Oneness. The living Tide dominates the awareness while forms move to the background. One feels the Breath of Creation in oneself as the Center of Wholeness. One feels the Unfoldment of oneself as one is Created. Our consciousness is a gift; we do not own it and if we try to control it we lose Wholeness.

Phase Nine is when we are able to fully evaluate and treat the Central Nervous System and the Eye. We also address Fire and the therapeutic modality of the Shakedown. True action is moved from Love and makes our perception exist. This Love is self-emptying and by its nature allows us to Serve as part of the Perfect. Perception can be used to Serve something other than ourselves. We have attempted to enter this balance point between the Perfect and the Disease ... it is a point where the whole of everything is suspended by Love as it works to incarnate the Complete. In the balance point of everything is The Intention of the Tide following the movement of the distortion back to a True relationship with the Blueprint of Life.

Pediatrics One explores how children grow as a whole, not in parts as we sometimes believe. Children live in the Direction of Ease of motion present in their fluid metabolic fields, otherwise they get uncomfortable and require assistance. Does your treatment directly support the whole, or does it assume to support the whole? We realize children are not adults and cannot be treated as adults are. We approach the therapeutic modality of the "Meeting Place", prenatal and postnatal periods, the treatment of the pelvis during pregnancy, fetal malposition and labor.

Pediatrics Two is where we deepen in the perceptive awareness necessary to approach the treatment of children. We deepen in our appreciation of Wholeness, the three levels of Stillness and the "Meeting Place". We approach "Desert Neutral", where therapeutics pass into the neutral substance, and a mystery unfolds as the breath of Divine love cascades as a therapeutic force across a night desert landscape, filling and leaving behind no visible effects. We further address treatment of the pelvis and the uterus during pregnancy. We explore thoracic and Primary Respiration in children, and the Family Circle.

Pediatrics Three is where we continue to study the therapeutic Flow of Attention. We deepen in Third Level Stillness and the Meeting Place. The Meeting Place is easily misinterpreted ... our observer must be so still and neutral that the process can be seen as it happens. The central nervous system in the child can be finally approached for evaluation and treatment. We explore teething and also the "locked up head". We use the therapeutic modality of the Flame of Intention, and its connection to the Breath of Life. Everything is transparent to the Breath of Life.

ABOUT THE AUTHOR

James Jealous, D.O. (1943–2021), was an osteopathic physician, teacher, and writer. His life's work was founding and developing **Biodynamics of Osteopathy**, a unique methodology he established within the field of osteopathy, following the lineage of Dr. A.T. Still and Dr. W.G. Sutherland.

He was born in Saco, Maine, and since his father was an osteopathic physician, he was around osteopathy from an early age. He studied at Kirksville College of Osteopathic Medicine in Missouri (now the A.T. Still University of Health Sciences), graduating in 1970. He then set up practice in rural Maine as an osteopathic primary care physician.

Over time, Dr. Jealous saw parallels between the work of embryologist Dr. Erich Blechschmidt and that of osteopathic physician Dr. William Garner Sutherland. This inspiration led him to create his own body of work. In the early 1990s, he began teaching "A Biodynamic View of Osteopathy in the Cranial Field," which, as he developed his specific methodology, was refined to "Biodynamics of Osteopathy."

A deeply spiritual person, he felt most at home in the natural world and was an avid fisherman and hiker.

For more information, please visit:
https://BiodynamicsOfOsteopathy.com

There is a wind passing through …
it is the motion of creation,
the eternal motion of Divine love.

www.ingramcontent.com/pod-product-compliance
Lightning Source LLC
LaVergne TN
LVHW071338210926
848486LV00003B/175

* 9 7 9 8 2 9 5 4 6 3 1 8 1 *